WITHDRAWN

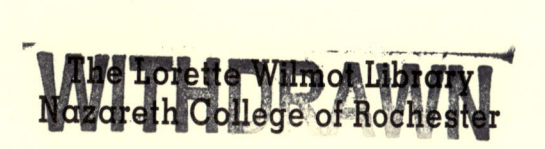

The Lorette Wilmot Library
Nazareth College of Rochester

DEMCO

A Sense of Direction

Activities to Build Functional Directional Skills

A Sense of Direction

Activities to Build Functional Directional Skills

by
Laura Sena

Foreword by
Ann Nolen

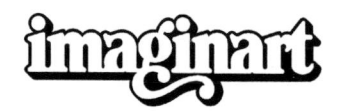

imaginart

Bisbee, Arizona

LORETTE WILMOT LIBRARY
NAZARETH COLLEGE

Imaginart International, Inc.
307 Arizona Street
Bisbee, AZ 85603

Phone: (800) 828-1376
(520) 432-5741
Fax: (800) 737-1376
(800) 432-5134
E-mail: imaginart@aol.com

Copyright © 1999 by Imaginart International, Inc. All rights reserved.

Permission is granted to reproduce the pages carrying the notice *"Reproducible. Copyright © 1999 Imaginart International, Inc."* in limited quantities for clinical use only. Other portions of this work may not be reproduced or transmitted in any form or by any means, including, but not limited to, electronic, mechanical, photocopying, and recording by any information storage or retrieval system without special permission from the publisher.

Edited by Cindy Drolet

Art Direction and Illustrations by Deborah Nore

Cover by Rick Menard

Library of Congress Cataloging-in-Publication Data

Sena, Laura, 1955-
    A sense of direction : activities to build functional directional skills / by
Laura Sena.
      p. cm.
    Includes bibliographical references.
    ISBN 1-883315-38-7 (pbk.)
    1. Orientation (Psychology)--Study and teaching (Elementary)--Activity programs.
I. Title.
BF299.07S46   1999
370. 15' 5--dc21
                                                                                             98-47876
                                                                                              CIP

Manufactured in the United States of America.

ISBN 1-883315-38-7

Dedication

To my family

Acknowledgment

I would like to acknowledge the influence of friend and colleague, Susan McDuffie, who contributed to the inception of this book.

Contents

Introduction 1

The Development of Directional Skills 3

    Body Awareness 3

    Postural Integration and Body Division 4

    Spatial Vision and Perception 6

    Left and Right Identification 6

    Higher Level Spatial Perception 8

    Summary 8

Perspectives on Disability and Directional Skills 11

Using A Sense of Direction 15

    Organization of Activities 15

    Assessment of Directional Skills 17

    Treatment Planning for Directional Confusion 18

    Goals and Objectives for Directional Skills 20

    Materials 20

    Optional Materials 21

Level 1 - Body Awareness 23

    Alligator 24

    Make-Believe Hospital 26

    Mud Bath 28

    Rolling Logs 30

    Where is the Sticker? 32

Level 2 - Self as a Reference Point 35

    Crumple 36

    Field Trip Marches 38

High 5's on all 4's...41

Keep Your Eye on the Ball..................................43

Leaning Tower...45

Left and Right Coin Sorting................................46

Tapping Patterns..48

Make-Believe Hospital (Modified for Level 2)...............50

Mud Bath (Modified for Level 2)............................52

Where is the Sticker? (Modified for Level 2)...............54

Level 3 - Environment as a Reference Point............57

More About Level 3 Activities..............................58

Two-Dimensional Space: Grid Map Games......................59

    Follow the Path..60

    Make a Map...70

    Park Your Penny..76

    Prairie Dog Town.......................................79

    Animal Parade..82

    Mixed-Up Socks...85

    Mail Delivery..88

    Secret Word..91

    Three-Ways Maze..94

    Secret Door..97

    File Cabinet..100

Three-Dimensional Space: Floor Grid Games and More........103

    Instructions for Making a Floor Grid..................104

    Using Floor Grids.....................................105

    Remote Control Robots.................................106

    Floor Grid Memory Match...............................108

    Sticker Hunt Floor Grid Game..........................118

    Animal Parade Floor Grid Game.........................120

    Mixed-Up Socks Floor Grid Game 126
    Mail Delivery Floor Grid Game..................... 132
    Secret Word Floor Grid Game 138
    Looking for Landmarks 140

Level 4 - Others as a Reference Point 143
    Paper People Cutouts 144
    Picture Poses..................................... 158
    Statue Maker...................................... 168
    Design a Pocket T-Shirt 170
    Follow the Path (Modified for Level 4) 174
    Make a Map (Modified for Level 4) 176
    Park Your Penny (Modified for Level 4) 178
    Three-Ways Maze (Modified for Level 4) 179

Fixed Reference Points 181

Games, Sports and Compensatory Strategies to Build
    Directional Skills............................. 183
    Games... 183
    Sports 184
    Compensatory Strategies........................... 185

Appendix 187
    Instructions for Quick Screen and Pre-/Post-Tests 188
    Quick Screen Test 190
    Pre-/Post-Tests 191
        Level 1—Body Awareness 191
        Level 2—Self as a Reference Point............. 192
        Level 3—Environment as a Reference Point..... 193
        Level 4—Others as a Reference Point 194
        Star Sheets 195
    Goals and Objectives 198

  Individual Planning and Progress Guide................200
  Sample Individual Planning and Progress Guide............202
  Blank Grid Maps 204
  Samples of Completed Grid Maps 209

Glossary 213

References 217

About the Author 221

Foreword

Growing up as a dancer I learned quickly that you had to know your right from your left or you didn't last very long in an activity dependent upon synchronized movement. I observed many aspiring classmates dropping out because they just couldn't get it. The frustration, embarrassment and discouragement they went through was only magnified when they were labeled as having "two left feet." Now, over 40 years later, Laura Sena, in *A Sense of Direction*, provides an understanding of why directionality, second nature to most, is a critical building block not only to fancy footwork but to everyday tasks.

Writing your name in the left-hand corner of the paper instead of the right-hand corner may be seemingly inconsequential, but turning the left faucet instead of the right when taking a shower could result in serious injury. As an occupational therapist with an impressive depth of clinical expertise, Laura Sena knows the magnitude of this problem and has the answer for clients who struggle with directional confusion and for clinicians who want to help them do something about it.

Fun, creative, imaginative and grounded in theory, this resource is a must for school-based occupational therapists, speech pathologists and teachers and will prove invaluable to others who seek to improve functional performance. Moreover, Sena, with her multi-level approach, has taken the guess work and worry out and provided the therapist with a compilation of 42 activities irresistible to children of all ages. From the new graduate to the seasoned therapist or teacher, this book has something for everyone—what you do, why you do it, how you do it and what to look for while you're doing it.

Ann H. Nolen, Psy.D., OTR
Assistant Professor
University of Tennessee, Memphis

Introduction

"Run out to left field."

"Turn east at the next intersection."

"Write your name in the upper left-hand corner."

"Go down the hall to the third door on your right."

These statements, though seemingly commonplace, reflect the omnipresence of direction in daily life. Our sense of direction grounds us and guides us. Its quiet presence reassures us and allows us to say "I know where I am."

Just as a strong sense of direction contributes to a feeling of security, directional confusion can result in fear and embarrassment. Who among us has never experienced the sinking feeling of disorientation? Recall times when you have traveled to a foreign city, learned a new dance step or searched for your car in the mall parking lot. Temporary directional confusion is a shared human experience.

For some people, however, directional confusion represents a pervasive problem that impedes functioning in daily life. The following excerpts from *Ann Landers* illustrate just how devastating directional confusion can be:

> **Dear Ann Landers:** I am swamped with work, but I just had to respond to the woman from Royal Oak, Mich., who is embarrassed because she has such a poor sense of direction. She is not the only one. I have been afflicted with this curse for as long as I can remember.
>
> I must allow an extra hour whenever I leave the house because it's a cinch I'll get lost, even though I have written instructions. No maps. They never work. The cell phone is on constantly. Sometimes, my husband will stay on the line for an hour giving me directions.
>
> My family and friends think it's funny, but it kills me to call from a neighboring city I've been to a hundred times and ask, "Which way do I turn to get home?" I feel like an idiot.
>
> *Pamella Iman*
> *Portland, Oregon*

Dear Ann Landers: I'm 54 now and have had a direction problem for as long as I can remember. When I was in elementary school, I would get lost coming back from the bathroom. I would never volunteer to go on an errand for the teacher because I knew I would never find my way back. Even now, I become totally disoriented when I'm a few blocks from home. I feel like a nitwit and it was extremely comforting to know I'm not alone.

Miami, Florida

Permission granted by Ann Landers and Creators Syndicate.

Clearly, directional confusion not only interferes with independence but also affects self-esteem. Adults struggling with these issues can usually trace their directional confusion back to childhood. The innate sense of direction that seemed to appear automatically in other children never developed in them. Instead, many children experiencing directional confusion grew up feeling inadequate and isolated, like those who wrote to Ann Landers.

A Sense of Direction was written to address this problem by helping children develop directional skills. Through carefully selected purposeful activities, children will experience, practice and learn spatial concepts. It is my hope that *A Sense of Direction* will contribute to a future of self-confidence and independence for those affected by directional confusion.

Laura Sena, OTR/L
Occupational Therapist
Registered and Licensed

The Development of Directional Skills

How does the sense of direction develop? What enables people to distinguish left from right? Why do some people become easily disoriented? Scientists have explored these questions since the turn of the century and, although their theories vary, they seem to share a common postulate: *body awareness* forms the basis for developing directional skills.

Body Awareness

From the very first days of life, the infant learns about his or her body through sensorimotor exploration. Piaget described this stage, from birth to about the age of two, as the sensorimotor period. The infant in the sensorimotor period learns about the environment as a result of sensory input and motor response to that input (Clark, 1985). By grasping, mouthing, rolling, crawling and creeping, the baby actively explores the world. The baby also interacts with objects and people in the environment. In so doing, the baby experiences many sensations coming from the outside world. With each new sensation, the baby makes a motor response, and, through experimentation, repetition and modification, learns new skills.

The baby also experiences sensations coming from inside the body. These sensations are generated by the baby's own movements. Perhaps the most powerful sensory information originating within the body comes from the vestibular-proprioceptive system. The vestibular and proprioceptive systems work in concert to play a vital role in the development of body awareness. The sensory receptors of the vestibular system, the otoliths of the inner ear, respond to gravity and changes in head position. Proprioceptors in the muscles and joints respond to changes in body position, weight bearing and movement. To understand these systems in action, envision a baby sitting on the floor. The baby sees her favorite toy and crawls to it on hands and knees. The baby activates vestibular and proprioceptive receptors when she turns her head and shifts her weight to her hands and knees. The movement of crawling toward the toy continues to activate the vestibular-proprioceptive system, giving the baby feedback about her body and the outside space through which she moves. Fisher, et al., in *Sensory Integration: Theory and Practice*, explain that this "vestibular-proprioceptive feedback from active movement contributes to the development of neuronal models," that is, "the memory of how it feels to perform a given movement" (1991, p. 91). It is through this feedback process that the vestibular-proprioceptive system provides a stable frame of reference against which other sensations are interpreted.

Among the other sensations that contribute to body awareness is touch. The tactile system encompasses the ability to interpret and discriminate light touch, pressure, temperature, pain and vibration. This information gives the growing baby very accurate feedback about her body. During the sensorimotor period, the baby also learns to locate objects in space with the help of vision and hearing. The baby will turn her head to find her mother's face or the sound of a ringing bell. The tactile, visual and auditory systems work together with the powerful vestibular-proprioceptive system to help the baby understand her body and her world. It is the culmination of this sensory information from both inside and outside the body, along with the adaptations the baby makes in response to those sensations, that results in body awareness.

The term *body awareness* actually encompasses three related components: body scheme, body image and body concept (de Quirós and Schrager, 1979).

By the age of two, the baby begins to organize sensory information into a *body scheme*. Body scheme is defined as "an internal awareness of the body and the relationship of body parts to each other"(American Occupational Therapy Association, 1994, p.13). As such, it is an internal map of the body to which the baby refers during activity (Parham and Mailloux, 1996).

This internal map of the body is expressed in the baby's growing ability to differentiate body parts. For example, when given a hat, the two-year-old readily places it on his head; during play he will hold a toy telephone up to his ear. A well-developed body scheme allows the baby to differentiate the top of his head from his ear in order to perform these tasks. Because body scheme is established on the cortical level, the two-year-old differentiates body parts automatically on an unconscious level.

Related to body scheme is the development of *body image*. The baby, with information about his body now organized into a schema, begins to develop a mental image of his body. The concept of body image encompasses more than the sensorimotor components of body scheme. Body image is thought to be the result of emotional and social influences as well as sensorimotor factors. Body image, therefore, changes from infancy to adulthood as the result of life experiences (de Quirós and Schrager, 1979).

As the growing baby's language skills emerge, *body concept* develops. When body concept is established, the baby not only recognizes body parts, but also identifies them by name. Thus, functional use of language is central in forming body concept.

Postural Integration and Body Division

By the age of three or four, sensory input from the vestibular, proprioceptive and visual systems coordinate to form an integrated postural system. This integration supports the development of more mature motor patterns in the toddler, allowing him to refine equilibrium responses, weight shifting and trunk rotation. At this stage of development, the toddler also begins to coordinate movements on different sides of his body (de Quirós and Schrager, 1979).

Body movement occurs relative to planes that divide the body into different sides. The body is divided into three planes of movement: *transverse, sagittal* and *frontal*. The transverse plane divides the body into top and bottom halves. The sagittal plane divides the body into left and right halves. Finally, the frontal plane divides the body into front and back halves. As the child experiences movement through these planes, he becomes increasingly aware that his body has different sides.

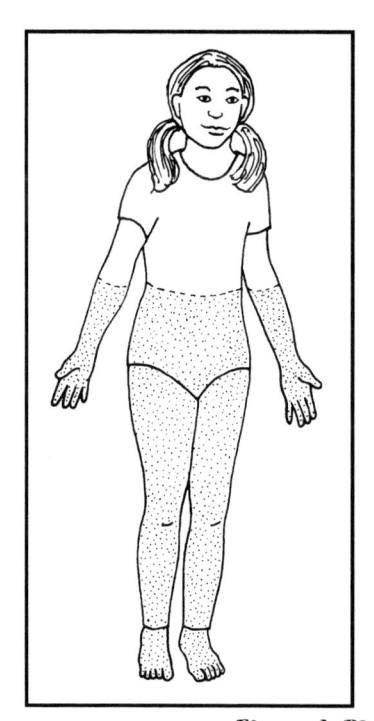

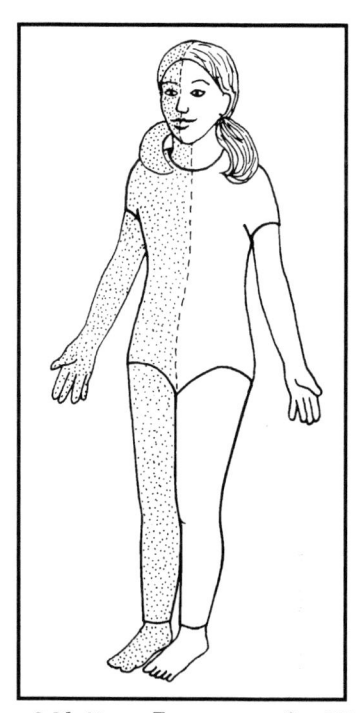

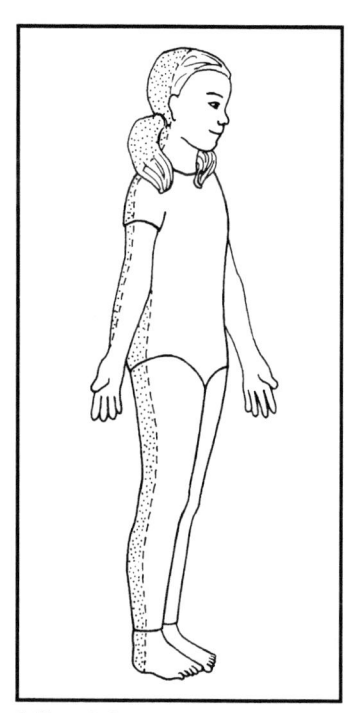

Figure 1: Planes of Motion—Transverse, Sagittal, and Frontal

As movement patterns mature, the left and right sides of the child's body learn to work separately until, by the age of four, specialized brain functions begin to lateralize. Murray explains that lateralization is the "process whereby hemispheres become specialized for a particular function; that is, a functional ability is said to be lateralized to one hemisphere or another" (1991, p. 174).

Between the ages of four and six, lateralization refines and the child has an internal awareness that her body has two sides. It is during this stage that hand preference may emerge. The child may consistently use her right hand to hold a spoon or reach for a cracker. Symbolic thought and language skills also develop and lateralize at this time. Motor responses are no longer driven by sensory input but are increasingly language directed.

Spatial Vision and Perception

It is important to recognize that while the growing child is developing body awareness, an integrated postural system, and lateralization—visual perception is also playing a role in the formation of directional skills. Visual perception gives meaning to what is seen. The component of visual perception that is most clearly associated with the development of directional skills is *spatial vision*. Schneck, in the third edition of *Occupational Therapy for Children,* explains that spatial vision "is concerned with the visual location of objects in space: where things are" (1996, p. 361).

As the growing child explores the world through sensorimotor experiences, he interacts with the environment to develop awareness of spatial concepts. Gradually, upon receiving sensory input, the child learns to differentiate, interpret and organize visual information into meaningful patterns of increasing complexity. This process, also described as *spatial perception,* is a complex and ongoing developmental process.

A synopsis of the early development of spatial skills, based on Gesell's developmental schedules (Knoblock and Passaminick, 1980) follows:

4-16 weeks	Ability to follow a moving object visually
36-56 weeks	Ability to place one cube in a cup on request
15-36 months	Ability to imitate a vertical stroke
18-36 months	Ability to place shapes into a formboard
24-36 months	Ability to imitate a horizontal stroke

36 months +	Ability to follow directions with prepositions–
	  on the chair
	  in front of the chair
	  in back of the chair
	  beside the chair

Left and Right Identification

By the age of five or six, an important milestone in the development of directional skills takes place: the child's sense of *left* and *right* appears. This ability occurs after the child has an internal awareness that his body has two sides. Hand dominance may also be established as a result of lateralization. The ability to recognize left and right is "established upon the continuity of body schema, body awareness and after the integration of the postural system"(de Quirós and Schrager, 1979, p. 40). As such, concepts of left and right are closely related to sensory information from within the body and, therefore, intrapersonal space.

The child's understanding of left and right matures gradually over several years. Initially, the child can only recognize left and right relative to her own body. A six-year-old, for example, may be able to identify her left ear or her right foot. In so doing, she is using herself as a reference point (intrapersonal space). As concepts of left and right become more automatic, she will learn to follow left and right instructions such as, "kick the ball with your left foot."

Gradually, a child learns to project spatial concepts originating from her own reference point to the outside world (extrapersonal space). She realizes that, like herself, objects have a left and a right side. For example, a place mat has a left and a right side; a baseball field has a left and a right field. As the child becomes skilled in understanding language concepts, she is capable of following more complex directions. For instance, she can follow instructions to "put the fork on the left side of the place mat" or "run out to right field." In these situations, the child uses the environment as a reference point.

Perceptual-motor theorists, most notably Cratty and Kephart, used the terms *laterality* and *directionality* to describe this stage of spatial skill development. According to perceptual-motor theory, *laterality* is an internal awareness that the body has a left and a right side. It is typically established by the age of six or seven. *Directionality* follows the development of laterality and emerges around the age of 8. It is the understanding that objects outside of the body also have a left and a right side (Schneck, 1996).

Another leap in directional skill development occurs when the child understands that each person views left and right from his own perspective. The child can recognize left and right not only in himself but also in other people—even those facing in the opposite direction. This requires a complex spatial operation whereby the child mentally rotates the position of left and right relative to himself and then projects it onto the person facing him. This high level skill is often necessary for giving directions to others such as, "As you walk down the hall, the bathroom will be on your right." It is also an important component of team sports such as soccer, basketball and football where opposing teams face one another and play field positions from their own left and right perspectives. During a football game, the defensive coach may tell his player to "Line up against the offensive right tackle." In these examples the individual must use others as a reference point to make spatial judgments.

The age at which these left and right directional skills emerge varies. Most researchers agree that the ability to recognize left and right on the self and follow simple left and right instructions relative to the self should be complete by the age of seven. Researchers vary in the chronology of developing an awareness of left and right in objects and understanding left and right in people facing in the opposite direction. Some note that understanding left and right in objects is the more complex skill, emerging around the age of eleven, while understanding left and right in people facing the opposite direction appears earlier, between eight and eleven years of age (de Quirós and Schrager, 1979). Others note that "the ability to identify right and left on people facing opposite directions can be confusing on into later childhood—and for some, into adulthood" (Levine, 1991, p. 507).

Higher Level Spatial Perception

In addition to refining and expanding concepts of left and right, the seven-year-old to twelve-year-old child is also developing higher level spatial skills. Among these are *position in space, spatial relations* and *topographical orientation*.

The development of *position in space* is complete at seven to nine years of age (Schneck, 1996). Position in space is the awareness of an object's position *relative to the self*. For example, the child may say, "The ball is behind my back." Position in space is important in using and understanding directional language concepts such as, in/out, up/down, in front/behind and left/right.

The development of *spatial relations* continues to improve until approximately ten years of age (Schneck, 1996). Spatial relations determine the position of objects *relative to each other*. The child shows an understanding of spatial relations when saying "The pencil is to the right of the magazine" or when following directions to build a model.

Topographical orientation emerges between the ages of six and seven but continues to develop through childhood and refine into adulthood. Through topographical orientation, the child determines the location of objects or destinations and the route needed to get there. A useful term used to describe this process is *wayfinding*. Wayfinding is a complex skill that involves several components operating concurrently. To walk from the cafeteria to the playground, for example, the child must have a cognitive map of the environment in place. A cognitive map includes "information about the destination, spatial information, instructions for execution of travel plans, recognizing places, keeping track of where one is while moving about, and anticipating features"(Schneck, 1996, p. 361).

Summary

In summary, the development of directional skills can be represented by the continuum shown in Table 1 on page 10. The development of directional skills begins with *body awareness* through sensorimotor exploration. Sensory information becomes *organized into a body schema* and its related components. It is from this schema or inner map of the body that the baby learns spatial concepts. As development proceeds with the maturation of an *integrated postural system* and *lateralization,* the growing child's understanding of spatial concepts also matures. This occurs initially in infancy through *spatial vision* as the baby learns to visually locate objects in space. As *spatial perception* develops, the child learns to discriminate and organize visual information by using the self as a reference point and later, by using the environment as a reference point. At this level the child's *sense of left and right* is established and *topographical orientation* emerges.

The continuum extends further as the older child develops *higher level spatial skills*. The child then learns to interpret spatial information for functional use through *spatial analysis* and *spatial planning*. Throughout the continuum, the child masters *spatial language concepts* to support and promote the development of directional skills. Directional skills continue to refine into adulthood.

Directional skills do not mature in isolation but concurrently with the development of body awareness, postural integration, lateralization, spatial perception and language. It is important to remember the vital role that active multisensory exploration and purposeful activity play in the development of these components. All of these elements are integrated to form a foundation for functional directional skills that will extend into adulthood.

Table 1. Development of Directional Skills

Age 0-2	Age 3-4	Age 4-6	Age 6-7	Age 7-12
Body Awareness through Sensorimotor Exploration	**Integrated Postural System** emergence of Coordination of Body Sides Relative to Body Planes	**Lateralization of Function** emergence of Hand Preference Symbolic Thought Language-Directed Actions	**Sense of Left and Right** established **Topographical Orientation** emerges	**Higher Level Spatial Skill Development**
Age 2 **Organization** into Body Schema Body Image Body Concept				

Concurrently Developing Skills

Spatial Vision → Spatial Perception → Spatial Analysis → Spatial Planning

Language Development

Table 1: Development of Directional Skills

Perspectives on Disability and Directional Skills

A child who has poor awareness of his own body and how it relates to extrapersonal space, does not have a strong foundation for building directional skills. He lacks a clear reference point from which to make spatial judgments. This weakness can manifest itself in the following ways in the school-aged child (Levine, 1991):

- left-right confusion
- difficulty following instructions with directional components
- frequently losing objects or becoming easily disoriented
- difficulty putting on clothing correctly
- poor organization of personal items or school materials
- avoidance of games, dances or sports
- difficulty comparing or estimating relative sizes and distances
- frequent reversals in reading and writing
- difficulty assembling puzzles or three-dimensional models
- frequently bumping into others or having difficulty staying in line with others

Directional confusion may result from a variety of causes. Neurological conditions such as minimal brain damage, traumatic brain injury, cerebral vascular accident or cerebral palsy may directly affect the brain's ability to process spatial information. Likewise, cognitive deficits resulting from disease or the aging process may impair neurological functions associated with direction sense. Physical disabilities restrict active sensorimotor exploration, thereby limiting opportunities to understand both intrapersonal and extrapersonal space during early development.

Other conditions, not directly associated with medical diagnoses, are also linked to weak spatial and directional skills. Among these is *sensory integrative dysfunction*. Sensory integration theory was developed by occupational therapist, A. Jean Ayres, out of her work with children who demonstrated sensorimotor or learning problems. Ayres postulates that children with sensory integrative dysfunction do not effectively organize and use sensory information. In a particular type of sensory integrative dysfunction called *somatodyspraxia*, children demonstrate poor body scheme development. Somatodyspraxia results from difficulty processing sensory information about body position, direction of movement and touch (Bundy and Koomar, 1991). Children with somatodyspraxia typically have difficulty with spatial relations and functional directional skills. They may also demonstrate problems with articulation and eating due to oral dyspraxia (Parham and Mailloux, 1996).

Researchers from the fields of educational psychology and behavioral optometry cite a strong correlation between spatial confusion and learning disability. Spatial knowledge is viewed as a prerequisite for reading and writing. Within this domain, deficits in visual discrimination and position in space clearly relate to problems with reading and writing such as letter reversals and poor spacing of writing on the page. Research has also been done linking left-right confusion to reading disability.

Clearly, there are strong associations between disability and directional confusion. Beyond theories linking directional confusion with specific disability, there exists a practical reality wherein directional confusion impedes daily life. A more effective way to discuss the ramifications of directional confusion, therefore, is to consider its impact on practical living skills. Consider how often direction sense comes into play on a typical day for the average adult:

> Upon rising you go to the bathroom to wash your face. You know without thinking which faucet handle to turn for hot water and which one to turn for cold water. You listen to the radio while you dress. You are concentrating more on the weather report than on how to dress, and yet you are able to quickly and automatically discern your left shoe from your right, the front of your shirt from the back, the top of your pants from the bottom. You set the table for breakfast. You put a plate on the center of a place mat. A fork goes to the left of the plate and a spoon to its right. You place your glass of juice in the upper-right-hand corner of the place mat. As you drive to work you encounter a detour for road repairs. You quickly plan an alternate route in your mind and still manage to get to work on time. You use a computer at work. Your left and right hands know where to go as you touch-type reports. You drag your computer mouse up, down, left and right to move through your document. After work you stop by the gym to exercise. You remember the left-right code to open your locker and change clothes. You attend a step aerobics class where the instructor introduces several new combinations. You admire her because she is facing the class while giving directional instructions—from the class' point of view. After dinner you sort and fold the laundry. You find time to organize your dresser drawers. For relaxation, you work on a needlepoint project, following a diagram. Finally, you go to sleep—on your favorite side of the bed.

The example described above illustrates the integral role direction sense has in daily life. More specifically, it demonstrates that by adulthood, direction sense is ingrained on an automatic level. Functional disability occurs when directional confusion interferes with independence in daily living skills. Directional confusion, therefore, should be addressed during early development and in the childhood years to most effectively improve functional skill.

Using A Sense of Direction

Optimal learning occurs during active participation in purposeful activity. *A Sense of Direction* includes 42 hands-on activities to build functional directional skills. The activities are based on a multisensory approach. Participants will move, touch, manipulate, visualize, speak, listen and draw to better understand spatial concepts. They will also learn strategies and compensatory skills to manage directional confusion.

Organization of Activities

The activities in *A Sense of Direction* are organized by level.

Level 1—Body Awareness

The activities in Level 1 enhance body awareness and facilitate the development of body scheme and body concept. A child participating in Level 1 activities will learn to differentiate and locate body parts in response to verbal request.

Level 2 - Self as a Reference Point

The activities in Level 2 focus on understanding directional concepts from the reference point of the self. A child participating in Level 2 activities will learn to differentiate directional concepts and follow directional instructions relative to himself.

Level 3 - Environment as a Reference Point

The activities in Level 3 promote an understanding of directional concepts relative to the environment. The environment is separated into two types of space—two-dimensional space (such as a piece of paper or a chalkboard) and three-dimensional space (such as a room or an object). A child participating in Level 3 activities will learn to differentiate directional concepts and follow directional instructions in both two- and three-dimensional space.

Level 4 - Others as a Reference Point

The activities in Level 4 build an understanding of directional concepts relative to the reference point of other people. During this level, a child will learn to differentiate directional concepts on others and give directional instructions to others.

The schematic in Table 2 depicts the levels of directional skill as steps beginning with Body Awareness at Level 1 and ending with Others as a Reference Point at Level 4. Note that as the steps progress, they follow a continuum from intrapersonal space to extrapersonal space. This reflects the growing child's ability to apply information learned in reference to the body, to objects and environments in the outside world.

Levels of Directional Skill

- **Level 1** — Body Awareness
- **Level 2** — Self as a Reference Point
- **Level 3** — Environment as a Reference Point
- **Level 4** — Others as a Reference Point

Intrapersonal Space ⟶ Extrapersonal Space

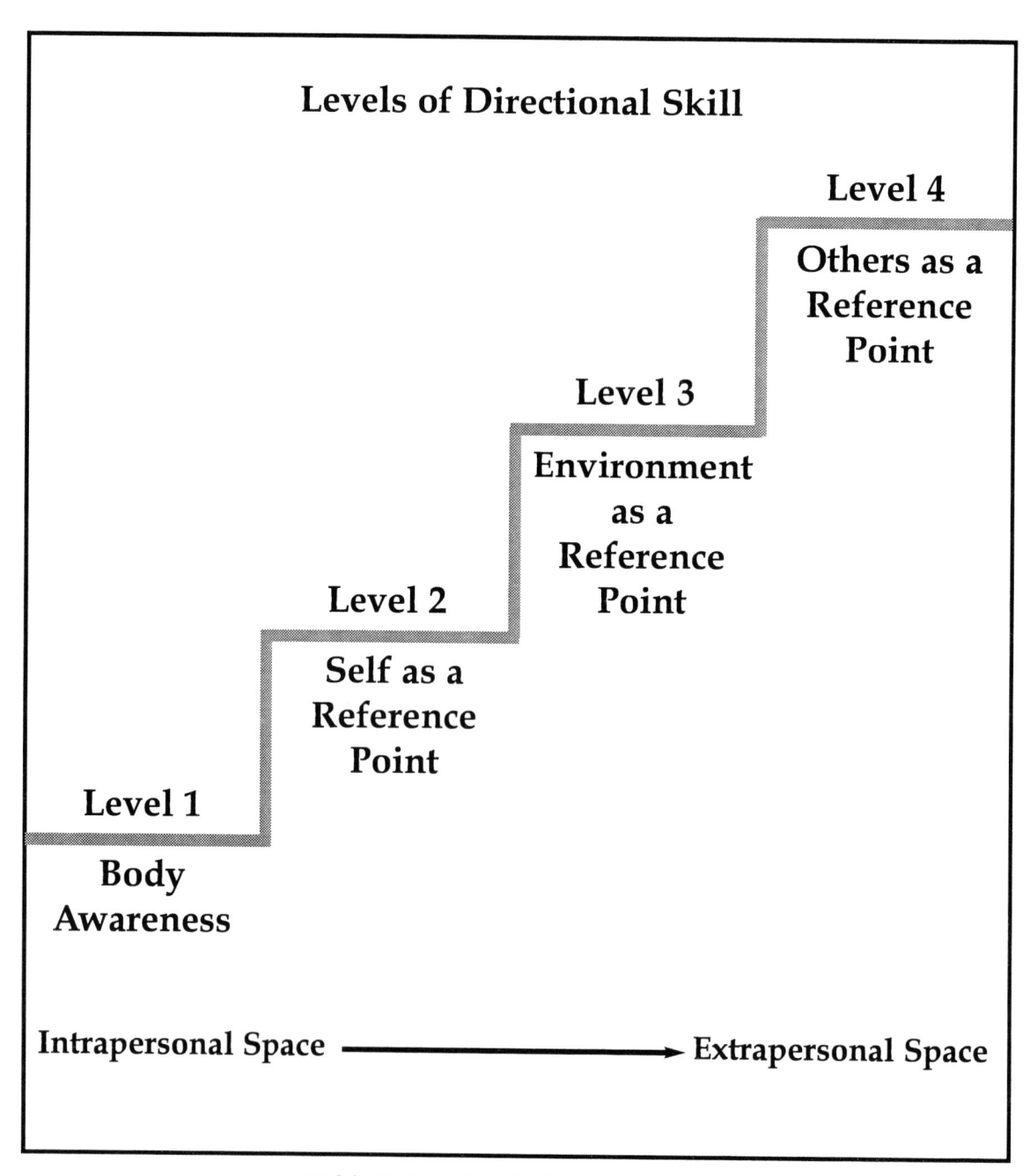

Table 2: Levels of Directional Skill

The following example helps illustrate the levels of directional skill:

Level 1

A very young child learns about her body through sensorimotor exploration. She has developed an inner sense of where her body parts are in relation to each other. When asked, she will readily point to her foot.

Level 2

As she matures, the child refines her understanding of spatial concepts. She is now aware that her body has a right and left, a front and back and a top and bottom. When asked, she will differentiate her right foot from her left foot.

Level 3

The growing child realizes that things and places outside of her body also have a left, right, front, back and so on. When given her shoes, she will be able to distinguish the left shoe from the right shoe and place each on the appropriate foot.

Level 4

As an older child, she understands that other people view directional concepts from their own perspective. She will be able to help her little brother put his shoes on the correct feet.

It is important to note that many of the activities in *A Sense of Direction* can be modified for multiple levels. This allows the instructor to use the same activity to target a higher level skill, thereby offering the participant new challenges.

Assessment of Directional Skills

In clinical studies, researchers have developed tests to assess spatial and directional skills. The most prevalent are tests of visual perception. Evaluation tools such as the *Test of Visual Perceptual Skills—(Non-Motor)* (Gardner, 1982) and the *Motor-Free Visual Perception Test-Revised* (Colarusso and Hammill, 1995) are commonly used by occupational therapists to screen for visual-perceptual dysfunction or to determine visual perceptual strengths and weaknesses. Though this information is helpful in assessing visual-perceptual processing, it does not yield data specifically about directional confusion. The *Jordan Left-Right Reversal Test* (Jordan, 1990) assesses visual reversal of letters, numbers and words. Other tests that evaluate directional skills as they relate to body awareness and body movement were developed by perceptual-motor theorists in the 1960s and 1970s; they are not listed among commonly used assessments by occupational therapists today (Asher, 1996). Among these are *The Purdue Perceptual–Motor*

Survey (Roach and Kephart, 1966) and the *Concepts of Left and Right Test* (Laurendau & Pinard, 1970). Occupational therapist, A. Jean Ayres, included a test of *Right-Left Discrimination (RLD)* in her battery, the *Southern California Sensory Integration Tests* (Ayres, 1979). This test is no longer included in the revised version titled the *Sensory Integration and Praxis Tests* (Ayres, 1989), although right-left confusion continues to be a clinical observation contributing to the assessment of sensory integrative dysfunction.

Formal assessment of directional skills is *not* necessary in order to use *A Sense of Direction*. In fact, observation and anecdotal reports by teachers and parents often give more valuable information about a child's functional directional skills. Upon referral, the practitioner can proceed with the standard assessment appropriate for the child and the setting (school system, private clinic, etc.). Standard assessments typically do not test a child's directional skills. The occupational therapy practitioner should, however, evaluate the developmental components affecting the acquisition of directional skills in the child. Among these components are: body awareness; bilateral integration; tactile, vestibular and proprioceptive processing. When deficits in these areas exist, the practitioner should determine if problems with directional skills are also present. Does the child confuse left and right? Does he have trouble following directional instructions? If problems such as these affect the child's functional performance in the home, school or community, further intervention is warranted. The first step of intervention is to determine the child's current level of directional skill.

A Sense of Direction includes a simple *Quick Screen* checklist to help determine a level of directional skill (see page 190). Accompanying the Quick Screen are *Pre- and Post-Test* checklists (pages 191-194). It is important to note that these checklists are *not* standardized, nor are the age ranges listed on the checklists based on empirical data. Rather, they are tools designed to approximate current level of function and track progress during treatment. The checklists are intended to be used along with the activities in *A Sense of Direction* at the discretion of the practitioner.

Treatment Planning for Directional Confusion

Therapy practitioners often face the dilemma of treating clients with multiple deficits in a limited time span. They must prioritize intervention according to need or urgency. Sometimes addressing directional skills as part of the treatment plan gets overlooked. Therapy practitioners can effectively incorporate directional skills into treatment plans. One way to accomplish this is to choose therapeutic activities that address concurrent performance components. By referring to the *Uniform Terminology for Occupational Therapy, Third Edition,* practitioners can determine which performance components to consider during assessment and intervention. These performance components "are the fundamental human abilities that–to varying degrees and in differing combinations–are required for successful engagement in performance areas (activities of daily living, work and productive activities, and play or leisure.)" (The American Occupational Therapy Association, Inc., 1994, p. 1). The following sensorimotor, cognitive and psychosocial performance components relate closely to spatial perception and direction sense:

- Sensory Awareness

- Sensory Processing—tactile, proprioceptive, vestibular, visual, auditory

- Perceptual Processing—stereognosis, kinesthesia, body scheme, right-left discrimination, form constancy, position in space, spatial relations, topographical orientation

- Motor—gross coordination, crossing the midline, laterality, bilateral integration, motor control, praxis, visual-motor integration

- Cognitive—memory, sequencing, categorization, concept formation, spatial operations, problem solving, learning, generalization

By carefully planning activities that incorporate the performance components above, the practitioner can facilitate the development of spatial perception and direction sense. Moreover, the therapy practitioner can incorporate directional skill development into a wide range of activities to address multiple deficits concurrently. Many activities in *A Sense of Direction* address concurrent deficits. An example of this is *High 5's on All 4's* (page 41). This is a Level 2 activity designed to help the child understand concepts of left and right relative to himself. In *High 5's on All 4's,* the child assumes a quadruped position facing the therapist. He then transitions into tall kneeling and, by reaching across midline with his left or right hand, lightly claps hands with the therapist. During this activity, the child learns to follow the practitioner's left and right instructions. But many other performance components are addressed concurrently. By weight bearing in the quadruped position, the child activates proprioceptive receptors. Transitioning into tall kneeling requires postural control and balance. Reaching across the body incorporates visual tracking, midline crossing, bilateral integration and praxis. Finally, through repetition, the child is learning and categorizing directional concepts.

In planning treatment to address directional confusion, the occupational therapy practitioner should be guided by these basic principles:

- Use active participation in meaningful tasks.

- Provide multisensory experiences to develop awareness of space and awareness of self in space (Levine, 1991).

- Provide opportunities to enhance vestibular-proprioceptive information.

- Perform active movements against resistance. This assists in the development of body scheme as a foundation for improving the planning of movement (Bundy and Koomar, 1991).
- Teach *specific* strategies. Strategies may include repetition, rehearsal, preplanning, visualization techniques and using multi-sensory cues to compensate for directional confusion.

Interdisciplinary collaboration is an effective way to incorporate *A Sense of Direction* into treatment. Although occupational therapy serves as the frame of reference for *A Sense of Direction*, other professionals such as speech-language pathologists and educators will find the program both pertinent and effective. The current trend in education is to share performance areas and goals with other team members when planning treatment for special needs children.

Keep in mind that, although the instructions in *A Sense of Direction* are written for one child, they can be easily adapted for groups. Practitioners working with adults who are developmentally disabled or individuals with cognitive impairments may find many of the activities suitable for their clients.

Goals and Objectives for Directional Skills

Writing goals and objectives is a difficult but mandatory requirement for all therapy practitioners. Although the format for writing goals and objectives may vary in different treatment settings, it is critical that they be specific and measurable. The authors of *OT Goals* (Aquaro, et al., 1992) recommend a format based on "who, what, how, where, and when" questions. Sample goals and objectives for developing directional skills based on this format are included in the appendix on pages 198-199. The samples present a variety of options for wording goals and objectives. Practitioners are encouraged to modify goals and objectives for the needs of their clients.

Accompanying the goals and objectives is a sample *Individual Planning and Progress Guide* (202-203). This guide allows practitioners working in school settings to refer to objectives as they plan activities for each nine-week quarter of the academic year. Practitioners working in other settings may modify the guide to meet their own needs.

Materials

The activities in *A Sense of Direction* were carefully designed to include only simple, readily available materials. Many of the activities also require worksheets which are provided as part of the manual for the practitioner to photocopy. The *A Sense of Direction* manual and all the materials for the program will easily fit into a canvas tote bag. Here is what you will need to start the program:

- 1 black marker
- pencils
- assorted colored pencils
- 3 wide point highlighting markers (pink, blue, yellow)
- 1 package of 100 blank index cards (4" x 6")
- 1 roll of masking tape (1" wide)
- tablet of lined paper
- small Post-it® Notes (1 1/2" x 2")
- scissors
- glue
- 10 pennies and 10 nickels in a small container
- 1 small ball
- several strips of stretchy fabric or assorted scarves and bandannas
- 1 rope (6' to 8' long)
- assorted small stickers (no larger than 3/4" x 3/4") available from

Mrs. Grossman's Stickers	PO Box 4467	Petaluma	CA	94955
Stickopotamus	PO Box 86	Carlstadt	NJ	07072
Sandylion Sticker Designs	PO Box 1570	Buffalo	NY	14240

Optional Materials

You will notice that at the end of each activity, there is a *More Ideas* section. Here you will find suggestions to expand the activity or combine it with other related tasks. You may need additional materials for the *More Ideas* section. The practitioner is encouraged to be creative and explore new ideas of her own.

Many of the activities in *A Sense of Direction* call for reproducible grid maps. If you prefer to reuse grid maps rather than make photocopies, you may modify the materials. To do this you will need sheet protectors and non-toxic, fine-point dry erase markers. Simply slide the grid map into the sheet protector and instruct the child to draw lines with the marker instead of a pencil. The child then traces the marker line with his finger. The dry erase marker line will magically disappear as the child traces.

Level 1—Body Awareness

Activities in Level 1 will help very young children become more aware of their bodies. Body awareness through active multisensory exploration promotes an inner sense of where body parts are in relationship to each other. Body awareness helps the child form a mental picture of the body.

Level 1 activities incorporate the vestibular-proprioceptive and tactile systems—shown to have a powerful influence in the development of body awareness. The activities in Level 1 focus on the ability to differentiate and locate body parts in response to verbal request. To complement the activities described in Level 1, children should be offered a variety of sensorimotor experiences providing vestibular-proprioceptive and tactile input during early development. Activity suggestions that can be planned into daily routines are listed below.

- Take babies out of play pens and walkers and allow sensorimotor exploration. **Remove potential safety hazards from the area and watch the baby at all times.**

- Name body parts while helping the toddler wash and dry at bath time. Use powder and lotion to give added tactile input to develop body awareness.

- Allow preschoolers to roll, tumble, jump and hang upside down.

- For indoor play, help preschoolers make hideouts. Use large boxes to climb in or tables covered with sheets to crawl under.

- Take preschoolers on frequent outings to the playground. Encourage climbing up and down on playground equipment, swinging and playing in the sandbox.

- Provide opportunities to play dress up. Include items for different body parts in the dress-up box such as belts, hats, gloves and jewelry as well as pants, shirts and dresses.

- Sing songs such as "Head, Shoulders, Knees and Toes" and finger plays such as "Where is Thumbkin?" to teach body part recognition.

Alligator

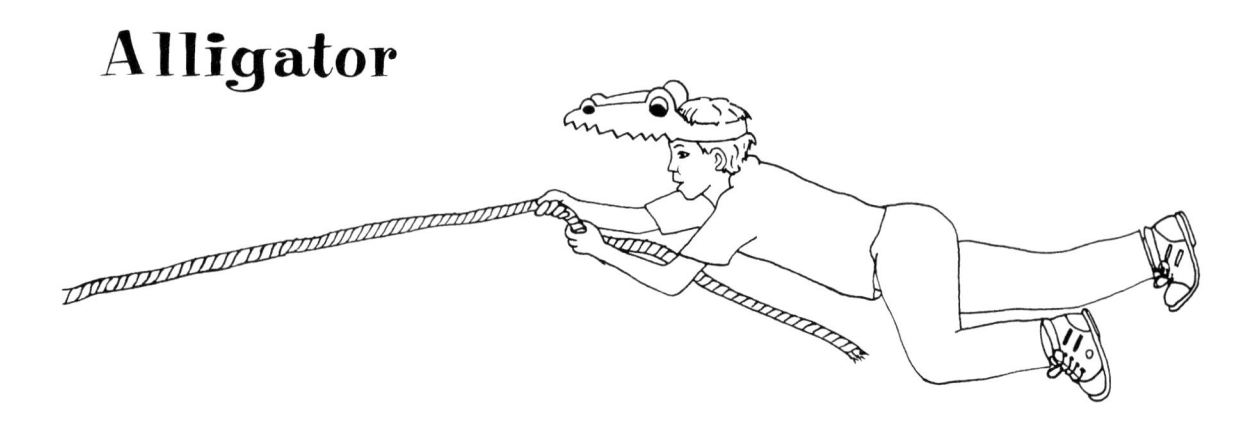

Purpose

To enhance basic body awareness through the vestibular-proprioceptive system. To promote use of both sides of the body. To facilitate the development of body scheme.

Materials

One rope (6' to 8' long)

Procedure

- Ask the child to be a "pretend alligator." Explain that alligators crawl on their stomachs. Ask the child, "Where is your stomach?"

- Place the rope on the floor and extend it across the room. Sit on the floor and hold one end of the rope. The "alligator" lies prone and holds the opposite end of the rope.

- Tell the child, "Pretend you are a *very* hungry alligator and that I have some delicious alligator food for you. Crawl on your stomach all the way to me. Use the rope to pull your body with your arms—first one arm then the other. Use your legs to push your body. Try to hold your alligator head up high."

- Reinforce the child and emphasize body awareness by saying, "You look like a real alligator crawling on your stomach. Your arms and legs are doing great work. I can see your alligator head!"

- When the child reaches you, give out the imaginary alligator food and repeat the game.

LEVEL I—BODY AWARENESS

- End the game by asking the child, "Show me your alligator stomach. Show me your alligator arms and legs. Show me your alligator head."

Observe

Can the child follow your instructions? Has he developed basic body awareness? Is the child learning to use both sides of the body in a smooth and coordinated way?

More Ideas

Using a picture of an alligator, discuss other body parts. Young children will want to imitate the alligator's big eyes and teeth. Compare and contrast other physical features by asking, "Do alligators have hands? Do people have tails? Do you think the alligator's skin is smooth like yours or rough and bumpy?"

Make-Believe Hospital

Purpose

To enhance body awareness through the tactile system. To facilitate the development of body scheme and body concept.

Materials

Several long strips of stretchy fabric or assorted scarves and bandannas

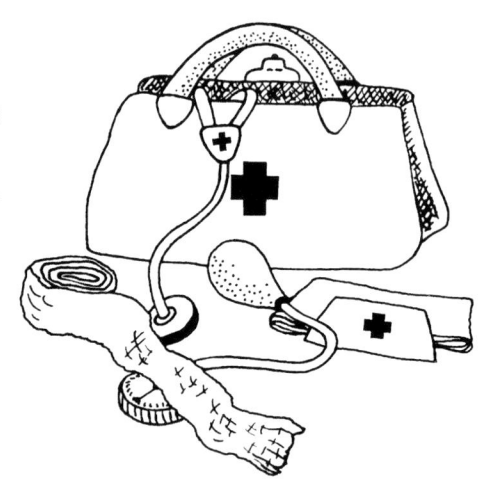

Procedure

- Explain to the child that you will be playing an imaginary hospital game. Discuss the difference between *real* and *make-believe* before starting the game.

- Tell the child, "Make-believe that you have hurt a body part. You can choose big body parts like your leg, arm, back, chest or head. Or, you can use smaller body parts like your elbow, ankle, knee, hand, foot or fingers."

- Continue instructing the child, "To start the game, tell me which body part is hurt. If you choose your thumb, say, 'Oh...I hurt my thumb!' Then show me where your thumb is by rubbing it."

- After the child has named and located the body part, wrap it with the fabric, taking care not to restrict circulation. Explain this step of the game by saying, "I will pretend to take care of your hurt body part by very carefully wrapping it in cloth. Keep the cloth on for a little while and remember where it is. Then I will take the cloth off and we will pretend that your hurt body part is healed."

- Repeat the sequence with other body parts. Assist the child if he cannot recall the name of a body part. Reinforce body awareness and body concept by talking to the child while you wrap the body part. Tell the child, "Oh, I see that you hurt your *thumb*. I will wrap your *thumb* with this cloth. Does your *thumb* feel better now?"

LEVEL I—BODY AWARENESS

- At the end of the game, have a "checkup." Tell the child, "I want to check if you can remember all the body parts I wrapped with the cloth. Tell me the name of the body part and show me where it is. I will help you if you can't remember."

Observe

Can the child name body parts accurately? Can the child locate body parts with ease? Has the child learned the names and locations of more complex body parts such as ankle, wrist, shoulder? Is the child uncomfortable when you wrap the body part? If so, he may be sensory defensive. If a child shows signs of discomfort, remove the cloth immediately.

More Ideas

You may want to expand this activity to discuss health and first aid. Invite a nurse or other medical professional to make a presentation appropriate for preschool-aged children. Include a toy doctor's kit in your setting.

Mud Bath

Purpose

To enhance body awareness through the tactile system. To facilitate the development of body scheme and body concept.

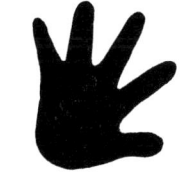

Materials

None

Procedure

- Sit on the floor with the child. Both you and the child roll up your shirt sleeves and pants. If you would like to, also remove shoes and socks.

- Tell the child, "We are going to have an imaginary mud bath. I have a great big bucket of cold, slimy mud here on the floor."

- Pretend to scoop mud from the imaginary bucket with your hands. Tell the child, "Watch me scrub my legs with mud. Now you scoop a big handful of mud from the bucket and scrub your legs. Try to look at your hands while you scrub."

- Repeat the sequence using various body parts. Carefully model the correct name and location of each body part for the child to imitate. Remember that you can put "mud" on many different body parts such as eyebrows, ears, lips, neck—you can even have a "mud shampoo."

- Next, place an imaginary bucket of water on the floor and say to the child, "We are covered with mud now. It's time to wash the mud off with this clean water."

- Ask the child, "Do you remember the names of the body parts we should wash? Which body part did we scrub with mud first? Tell me the name of the body part and show me where it is. Then you can pretend to wash the mud off with the water."

Observe

Can the child name body parts accurately? Can the child locate body parts with ease? Can the child remember the body parts in correct sequence? Notice how the child "scrubs" the body part with his or her hands. Are the hand movements slow and awkward or brisk and confident? Does the child visually attend to the task?

More Ideas

Provide a dry wash cloth for the child when it is time to "wash the mud off with clean water." Or try a sponge, surgical scrub brush or pre-moistened towels. The new texture will provide a different kind of tactile input to reinforce body awareness.

LEVEL 1—BODY AWARENESS

Rolling Logs

Purpose

To enhance basic body awareness through the vestibular-proprioceptive system.

Materials

A carpeted floor or a gym mat

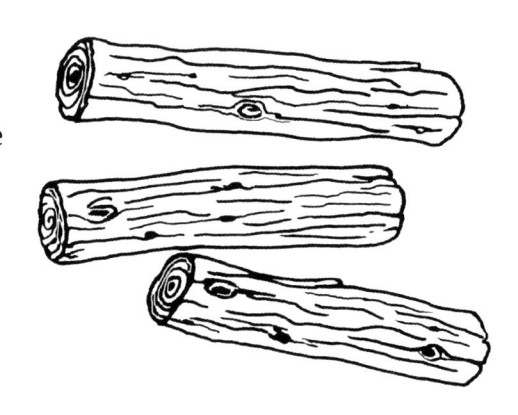

Procedure

- Ask the child to pretend to be a log of wood. Tell the child, "Lie on your back so that you can see the ceiling. Keep your body straight and stiff like a log. Squeeze your legs together so your feet touch each other. Keep your arms at your side."

- Tell the child, "Right now you are lying on your back. Can you feel your back pressing against the floor? Now log roll over onto your stomach. Are you looking at the floor? Can you feel your stomach press against the floor? Now log roll again so that you are on your back, looking at the ceiling like before."

- Continue instructing the child as follows. "I will tell you to roll by saying 'go' or 'stop.' You can roll in any direction you want. Sometimes when you stop you will be on your *back*. Sometimes when you stop you will be on your *stomach*. When you stop, tell me if you are on your back or stomach."

- Call out "go" and watch the child roll. Time your verbal cue to "stop" so that the child will be lying on his stomach. Then ask the child, "Are you on your back or your stomach?" After his response, continue the sequence and this time say "stop" when the child is lying on his back. Continue the sequence, varying the ending position.

Observe

Can the child follow your directions? Does the child understand the difference between lying on the back and lying on the stomach? Notice the rolling pattern. Can the child roll smoothly keeping the body straight?

More Ideas

When the child understands the difference between lying on the back and lying on the stomach, you may vary the game to make it more challenging. Instead of saying "go" and "stop," say "go" and "stomach" or "go" and "back." When the child hears the word *stomach,* he must stop on his stomach. When the child hears the word *back,* he must stop on his back.

Where is the Sticker?

Purpose

To enhance body awareness through the tactile system. To facilitate the development of body scheme and body concept.

Materials

A variety of stickers

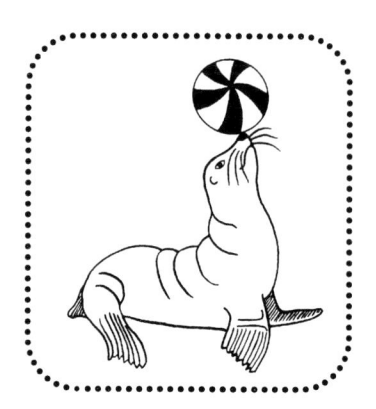

Procedure

- Explain that you will be playing a game using the sense of touch. Allow the child to choose a sticker.

- Tell the child, "I am going to put the sticker somewhere on your body. I might put it on your back, shoulder, elbow, wrist, hand or knee. If you keep your eyes closed and concentrate, you will be able to feel where I put the sticker."

- Instruct the child to close her eyes. Place the sticker on a body part, making sure to apply enough pressure for the child to sense the sticker's location.

- Ask the child, "Where is the sticker?" Allow the child to open her eyes to locate the sticker, then ask, "What is that body part called?"

- Ask the child to remove the sticker. Tell the child, "Try to remember this sticker and where it was. I will show it to you again at the end of the game."

- Continue the game using new stickers and different body parts. Ask the child to remember each sticker and its location on the body.

- At the end of the game, take out all of the stickers. Ask the child, "Do you remember these stickers? Which sticker was the very first one we used? Do you remember where it was? Can you say the name of the body part it was stuck on?" The child gets to keep all of the stickers that she recalls correctly.

LEVEL I—BODY AWARENESS

Observe

Can the child locate and name the body parts? Can she recall the stickers that correspond to the body parts? Does the child show signs of tactile defensiveness or is she comfortable with the activity?

More Ideas

Make this game more challenging by requiring the child to keep her eyes closed when naming the location of the body part.

Level 2—Self as a Reference Point

The activities in Level 2 will help children understand directional concepts within their own bodies. At this level, children have developed body scheme and body concept. They are now learning that their body has different sides: a top and bottom, a front and back and a left and right. When they have a clear understanding of these concepts, they can learn to follow instructions that have directional components such as, "Raise your right hand" or "Touch the top of your head." These spatial judgments are made from the point of view of the child. As such, Level 2 skills relate to intrapersonal space.

There are many everyday examples of Level 2 skills. Among them are shaking hands, making the Pledge of Allegiance and playing games such as Simon Says, Hokey-Pokey, Mother May I and Twister.

The activities in Level 2 focus on the ability to differentiate directional concepts and follow directional instructions relative to the self. Directional concepts and instructions included are right/left, top/bottom, front/back, up/down, forward/backward and above/below.

Please note that some of the activities in this level are modified from the Level 1 activities. Modifying previous activities allows reinforcement through repetition, but at a higher level of challenge. Children will enjoy learning new skills by repeating their favorite games that have been modified.

Crumple

Purpose

To reinforce body scheme and body concept. To differentiate directional concepts relative to the self.

Materials

Chair, blindfold and one piece of paper

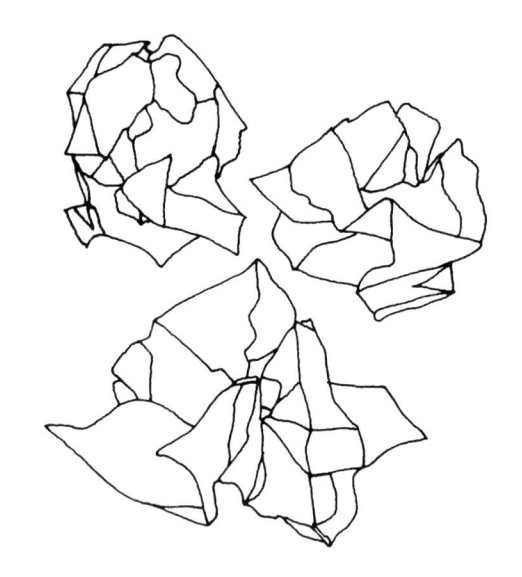

Procedure

- Ask the child to sit on the chair. Explain that you will be playing a listening game.

- Tell the child to *watch* and *listen* as you crumple the piece of paper. Say, "I am going to crumple this piece of paper. Do you hear the sound that it makes?"

- Allow the child to crumple the paper to hear the sound it makes. Say, "Now you crumple the piece of paper. Try to remember the crumpling sound that the paper makes."

- Cover the child's eyes with the blindfold. Instruct her to sit very quietly and listen for the crumpling sound.

- Tell the child, "I am going make the crumpling sound now. You try to guess *where* the crumpling sound is coming from. You might hear it on your right or left, in front of you or in back of you, above you or below you."

- Hold the paper in different positions and make the crumpling sound. In each position say, "Tell me where the sound is." After the child responds, remove the blindfold so that she can see the location of the paper.

- Continue the sequence, varying the location of the sound.

LEVEL 2—SELF AS A REFERENCE POINT

Observe

Has the child developed body awareness and body scheme? Can the child differentiate directional concepts on herself? Are the child's responses quick and automatic, or is there a noticeable delay in response time? Is the child able to screen out distractions and sit quietly to focus on the auditory input?

More Ideas

Vary the activity by using other sounds, for example, a ringing bell, scraping sandpaper or tapping pencils.

Field Trip Marches

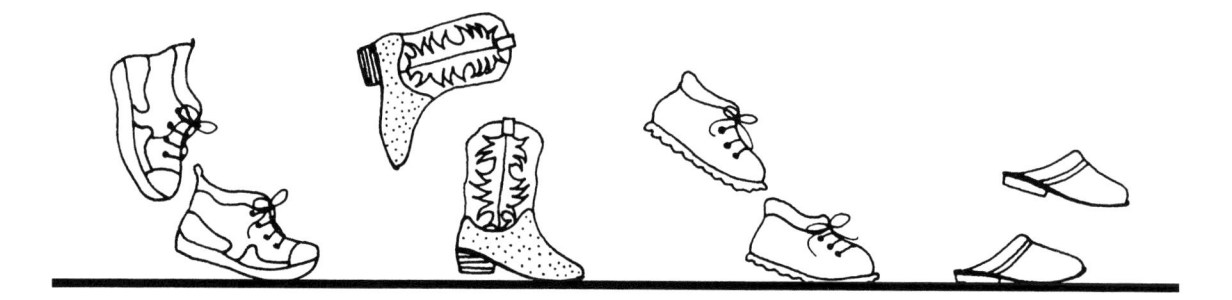

Purpose

To reinforce body scheme and body concept. To differentiate left and right relative to the self. To promote the ability to follow left and right instructions relative to the self.

Materials

None

Procedure

- When going on a walking field trip, instruct the child to follow the left and right instructions of a marching song.

- Allow the child to watch and listen as you model accurate left and right steps in sequence with the marching song.

- Tell the child, "Now let's march together. Get your left foot ready." Proceed with a left, right marching cadence. Encourage the child to say the marching song along with you.

Observe

Can the child follow the rhythm of the cadence? Does he use the correct foot? Can the child talk and march at the same time? On the next page is an example of a marching song (or cadence) that I learned at Girl Scout Camp:

Gingerbread

Left
Left
Left, right, left.
I left my wife with 48 children
Alone in the kitchen
In starving condition
without any gingerbread...
Left
Left
Left, right, left.

Here are two other cadences that your students may enjoy:

Up One Mountain

(Start Left)
Up one mountain
Down another
I can climb them
Like no other
Left
Left
Left, right, left
Left
Left
Left, right, left

Across one valley
Into another
I can hike them
Like no other
Left
Left
Left, right, left
Left
Left
Left, right, left

Through one cave
And out another
I can search them
Like no other
Left
Left
Left, right, left
Left
Left
Left, right, left

Climb one tree
Swing to another
I can climb them
Like no other
Left
Left
Left, right, left
Left
Left
Left, right, left

Source: Original cadence by Sunshine Echevarria. Used with permission.

LEVEL 2—SELF AS A REFERENCE POINT

Wash the Dishes

(Start Left)
Wash the dishes
Sweep the floor
Don't want to clean up
Anymore
Left,
Left,
Left, right, left

Source: Original cadence by Sunshine Echevarria. Used with permission.

More Ideas

Use opportunities to practice left/right marches during everyday situations, such as walking from the classroom to the cafeteria or taking the dog for a walk around the block.

Ask children to make up their own left/right marches—the sillier, the better.

High 5's on All 4's

Purpose

To reinforce body scheme and body concept. To differentiate left and right relative to the self. To follow left and right instructions relative to the self.

Materials

Carpeted floor

Procedure

- You and the child get in a quadruped position (on hands and knees) on the floor and face each other.

- Together, you move from quadruped to a tall-kneeling position. Tell the child, "Kneel up with me. Try to keep your balance so you kneel up straight and tall."

- Hold up your right hand. Tell the child, "I will call out 'right.' You reach across your body and give me a *high 5* with your *right* hand. Then we will both go back to the hands and knees position."

- Hold your left hand up and say, "Kneel up again. This time reach across your body and give me a *high 5* with your *left* hand, then return to hands and knees like before."

- Tell the child, "To continue the game, listen to my instructions. Sometimes I will call out 'left' and sometimes I will call out 'right.' Remember to use the hand that I name."

Observe

Is the child able to differentiate left from right? Can the child follow your left and right instructions?

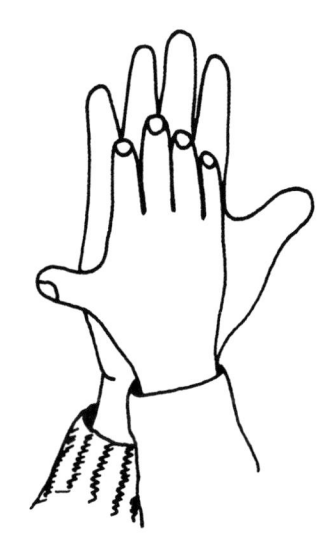

LEVEL 2—SELF AS A REFERENCE POINT

More Ideas

Besides directional skills, use this activity to develop postural control, equilibrium, bilateral integration, midline crossing and visual tracking.

Keep Your Eye on the Ball

Purpose

To differentiate left and right relative to the self. To follow left and right instructions relative to the self.

Materials

Table, chairs, masking tape and a small ball

Procedure

- Use the masking tape to divide the table in half. You and the child sit on opposite sides of the table with the masking tape aligned at midline.

- Tell the child, "Put your right hand on the table and your left hand in your lap. I will call out 'right,' and I will roll the ball to your *right* hand. Use your right hand to roll the ball back to me." Repeat several times.

- Continue instructions by saying, "Now put your left hand on the table and your right hand in you lap. This time I will call out 'left,' and I will roll the ball to your *left* hand. Use your left hand to roll the ball back to me." Repeat several times.

- Tell the child, "Now put both hands on the table. When I roll the ball to you I will call out 'left' or 'right.' Use the hand that I call out to roll the ball back to me. You may have to reach across the tape to roll the ball with the correct hand."

- Continue the game, varying the left and right instructions. Also, vary the *location* of the ball so that the child will have to reach across the tape line to return it to you some of the time. Make sure that you give the left and right instructions from the reference point of the child. Remind the child: "Keep your eye on the ball."

Observe

Is the child able to differentiate left from right automatically? Can the child follow your left and right instructions consistently?

LEVEL 2—SELF AS A REFERENCE POINT

More Ideas

Use this activity to build other skills such as visual tracking, visual-motor coordination, bilateral motor coordination and midline crossing.

Try using different types of balls: tennis balls, ping-pong balls, Nerf balls, hand balls and glide balls. You will find that each type of ball moves in a unique way.

Remove the masking tape from the table and speed up the game to increase the level of difficulty.

Leaning Tower

Purpose

To reinforce body scheme and body concept. To differentiate directional concepts relative to the self.

Materials

One firm cushion or pillow

Procedure

- Place the cushion on the floor. Ask the child to stand on the cushion facing you with shoes off.

- With your thumbs pointed up say, "Hold onto my thumbs." Then wrap the rest of your fingers around the child's hand for support.

- Tell the child, "Pretend that you are a tall, stiff tower. Keep your hips and shoulders steady. Try to balance on the cushion while I make you lean. Don't let go of my thumbs."

- Using your arms, push and pull the child slightly off center in different directions. Tell the child, "I am going to make you lean in different directions. I will tell you which way you are going—forward, backward, left or right. Try to say the words with me."

- Continue instructing the child by saying, "Now you tell me which way you are leaning all by yourself. Are you going forward, backward, left or right?"

Observe

Can the child differentiate directional concepts? Are the child's responses automatic or delayed?

More Ideas

Use this activity to improve proximal stability, postural control and equilibrium reactions. Try using a balance disc or tilt board.

Left and Right Coin Sorting

Purpose

To differentiate left and right relative to the self. To follow left and right instructions relative to the self.

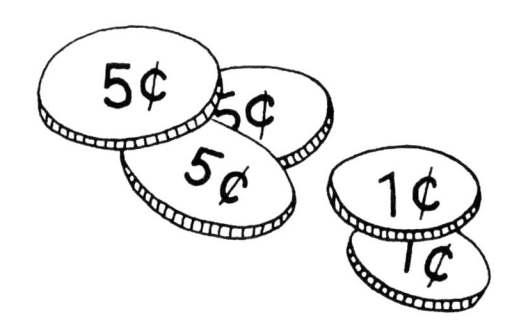

Materials

Ten pennies, ten nickels and an empty container

Procedure

- Mix up the pennies and nickels and spread them on the floor. Place the empty container nearby.

- Tell the child, "This is a game to help you remember left and right. Use your left hand to pick up all the pennies and your right hand to pick up all the nickels."

- Continue instructing the child by saying, "Try to pick up the coins one-by-one and put them into the container as fast as you can. When you pick up a penny say 'left'; when you pick up a nickel say 'right.' If you have trouble saying the left and right words, I will help you."

- Say "go" to start the game.

Observe

Can the child differentiate left and right? Does the child have difficulty remembering which hand picks up the penny and which hand picks up the nickel? If so, try taping a penny on the back of the left hand and a nickel on the back of the right hand.

More Ideas

Use this activity to develop fine motor dexterity, bilateral motor coordination and sorting.

LEVEL 2—SELF AS A REFERENCE POINT

Combine this activity with a math unit on money using different sets of coins. After the game, have the child count the coins and add up the total. Use a stopwatch to time the child. Repeat the game and encourage the child to beat his own time record.

Tapping Patterns

Purpose

To differentiate left and right relative to the self. To follow left and right instructions relative to the self.

Materials

Table and chairs

Procedure

- Sit next to the child so that you are facing in the same direction.
- Tell the child, "Watch and listen carefully as I tap my hand on the table. I will use my right hand first."
- Use your right hand to tap slowly three times. Say "right, right, right" as you tap.
- Ask the child to imitate your pattern by saying, "Now you tap three times with your right hand. Say 'right, right, right' as you tap."
- Continue instructing the child by saying, "I will make more tapping patterns. Sometimes I will use my right hand and sometimes I will use my left hand. Watch and listen to my pattern, then try to copy me. Remember to say the left and right words as you tap. I will say the words with you if you need help."
- Proceed by making left and right tapping patterns on the table for the child to imitate. Tap slowly and deliberately. Try different left and right combinations.

Observe

Can the child differentiate left and right? Can the child say "left" or "right" while tapping? Can the child remember the tapping pattern?

More Ideas

Use this activity to develop bilateral motor coordination, motor planning, listening and sequencing skills.

If the child has difficulty, provide a sensory cue by putting stickers with an "L" and an "R" on the back of the child's hands. Ideas for other cues include wearing a wrist weight, bracelet or ring to distinguish one hand from the other.

Increase the level of difficulty by lengthening the pattern.

Allow the child to make up a pattern for you to copy.

Note

The next group of activities are modified from Level 1 to address Level 2 skills. You may want to refer back to the Level 1 descriptions under the same activity names.

Make-Believe Hospital
Modified for Level 2

Purpose

To reinforce body scheme and body concept. To differentiate left and right body parts relative to the self.

Materials

Several long strips of stretchy fabric or assorted scarves and bandannas

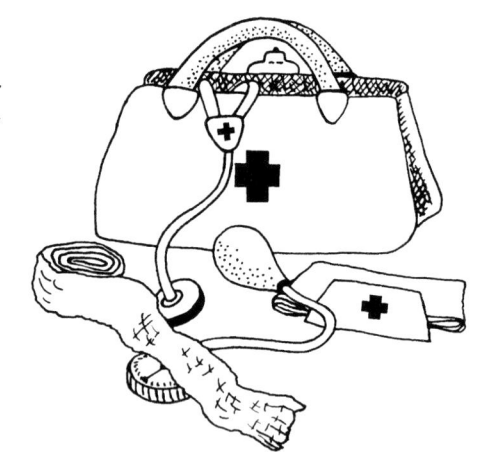

Procedure

- Explain to the child that you will be playing an imaginary hospital game. Discuss the difference between *real* and *make-believe* before starting the game.

- Tell the child, "Make-believe that you have hurt a body part. Choose a body part that has a left and a right such as, a shoulder, elbow, wrist, hand, knee or ankle."

- Continue instructing the child, "To start the game, tell me which left or right body part is hurt. If you choose your right elbow, for example, say 'Oh...I hurt my *right* elbow!' Then show me where your *right* elbow is by rubbing it."

- After the child has named and located the left or right body part, wrap it with the fabric, taking care not to restrict circulation. Explain this step of the game by saying, "I will pretend to take care of your hurt body part by very carefully wrapping it in cloth. Keep the cloth on for a little while and remember where it is. Then I will take the cloth off, and we will pretend that your hurt body part is healed."

- Repeat the sequence with other left and right body parts. Assist the child if he cannot recall the name of a body part. Reinforce body scheme and body concept by talking to the child while you wrap the body part. Tell the child, "Oh, I see that you hurt your *right* elbow. I will wrap your *right* elbow with this cloth. Does your *right* elbow feel better now?"

LEVEL 2—SELF AS A REFERENCE POINT

- At the end of the game, have a "Left and Right Checkup." Tell the child, "I want to check if you can remember all the left and right body parts I wrapped with the cloth. Tell me the name of the body part and show me where it is. I will help you if you can't remember."

Observe

Can the child locate and differentiate left and right body parts accurately? Is the child uncomfortable when you wrap the body part? If so, he may be sensory defensive. If a child shows signs of discomfort, remove the cloth immediately.

More Ideas

You may want to expand this activity to discuss health and first aid. Invite a nurse or other medical professional to make a presentation appropriate for children.

Mud Bath
Modified for Level 2

Purpose

To reinforce body scheme and body concept. To differentiate left and right relative to the self. To follow left and right instructions relative to the self.

Materials

None

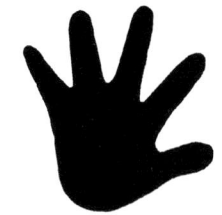

Procedure

- Sit on the floor next to the child so that you are facing the same direction. Both you and the child roll up your shirt sleeves and pants. If you would like to, also remove shoes and socks.

- Tell the child, "We are going to have an imaginary mud bath. I have a great big bucket of cold, slimy 'mud' here on the floor."

- Pretend to scoop mud from the imaginary bucket with your hands. Tell the child, "I am going to scrub a left or right body part with mud. Watch me scrub my *left* leg with mud. Now you scoop a big handful of mud from the bucket and scrub your *left* leg. Try to look at your hands while you scrub."

- Repeat the sequence using various left and right body parts. Carefully model the correct name and location of each body part for the child to imitate. Remember that you can put "mud" on many different left and right body parts such as eyebrows and ears.

- Next, place an imaginary bucket of water on the floor and say to the child, "We are covered with mud now. It's time to wash the mud off with this clean water."

- Ask the child, "Do you remember the left and right body parts we washed? Which body part did we scrub first? Tell me the name of the body part and show me where it is. Remember to tell me if it is a left or a right body part. Then you can pretend to wash the mud off with water."

LEVEL 2—SELF AS A REFERENCE POINT

Observe

Can the child locate and differentiate the left and right body parts accurately? Can the child remember them in correct sequence? Notice how the child "scrubs" the body parts with his hands. Are the hand movements slow and awkward or brisk and confident? Does he visually attend to the task?

More Ideas

Provide a washcloth for the child when it is time to "wash the mud off with clean water." Or try a sponge, surgical scrub brush or pre-moistened towels.

Try using other directional concepts for this activity such as the top of your head, bottom of your foot, in between your fingers, under your chin, etc.

LEVEL 2—SELF AS A REFERENCE POINT

Where is the Sticker?
Modified for Level 2

Purpose

To reinforce body scheme and body concept.
To differentiate left and right relative to the self.

Materials

A variety of stickers

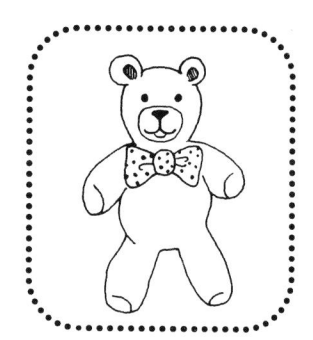

Procedure

- Explain that you will be playing a game using the sense of touch. Allow the child to choose a sticker.

- Tell the child, "I am going to put the sticker somewhere on your body. I will put it on a left or right body part such as your shoulder, elbow, wrist, hand or knee. If you keep your eyes closed and concentrate, you will be able to **feel** where I put the sticker. Try to decide if it is a left or a right body part."

- Instruct the child to close her eyes. Place the sticker on a left or right body part, making sure to apply enough pressure for the child to sense the sticker's location.

- Ask the child, "Where is the sticker?" Allow the child to open her eyes to locate the sticker. Then ask, "What is that body part called? Is it left or right?"

- Ask the child to remove the sticker. Tell the child, "Try to remember this sticker and where it was. I will show it to you again at the end of the game."

- Continue the game using new stickers and different left and right body parts. Ask the child to remember each sticker and its location on the body.

- At the end of the game, take out all of the stickers. Ask the child, "Do you remember these stickers? Which sticker was the very first one we used? Do you remember where it was? Can you say the name of the left or right body part it was stuck on?"

LEVEL 2—SELF AS A REFERENCE POINT

- Allow the child to keep all of the stickers that she recalls correctly.

Observe

Can the child locate and differentiate the left and right body parts? Can she recall the stickers that correspond to the body parts? Does the child show signs of tactile defensiveness, or is the child comfortable with the activity?

More Ideas

Make this game more challenging by requiring the child to keep her eyes closed when naming the location of the left or right body part.

Level 3—Environment as a Reference Point

The activities in Level 3 will help children understand directional concepts in the outside world. At this level, children already understand that their bodies have different sides. They are able to differentiate directional concepts on themselves and follow directional instructions relative to themselves. They are now ready to learn that, like themselves, objects and settings in the environment have a left and right, front and back and top and bottom. They will learn to project directional concepts from their own bodies onto objects and settings in the environment. They will learn to make spatial judgments from a point of view outside of their bodies. As such, Level 3 skills relate to extrapersonal space.

Extrapersonal space can be categorized into *two-dimensional space* and *three-dimensional space*. Flat surfaces take up two-dimensional space. Examples of surfaces in two-dimensional space are chalkboards, computer screens, pieces of paper, maps and newspapers. Flat surfaces have a left and right, front and back, top and bottom and center. Objects and settings in the environment take up three-dimensional space. Examples of objects and settings in three-dimensional space are a block, a shoe, a file cabinet, a baseball field, a classroom and a grocery store. Objects and settings in three-dimensional space have a left and right, front and back, top and bottom and center.

The following are some everyday examples of Level 3 skills.

Two-Dimensional Space	**Three-Dimensional Space**
Writing your name in the upper right-hand corner	Going to the back of the line
Reading the footnote at the bottom of the page	Looking in the drawer on the right
Scrolling down the computer screen	Putting a box on the top shelf

The activities in Level 3 focus on the ability to differentiate directional concepts and follow directional instructions in both two- and three-dimensional space. Directional concepts and instructions included are right/left, top/bottom, front/back, up/down and forward/backward.

Please note that some of the activities in this level are modified from the

Level 2 activities. Modifying previous activities allows reinforcement through repetition, but at a higher level of challenge.

More About Level 3 Activities

Most of the activities in Level 3 are based on a *grid system*. A grid is a series of vertical and horizontal lines serving as directional coordinates. For these activities, the purpose of the grid is to help children orient themselves in space. Children will refer to the grids to move left, right, up, down, forward or backward. There is *no* diagonal movement in the grid. The activities require two-dimensional space grids, three-dimensional space grids or both.

You will use paper grid maps for two-dimensional space activities. Reproducible grid maps are included for each two-dimensional space activity. For some of the activities, you will need to save the completed grid map for use in a floor grid game. Children will draw during grid map games. These activities, therefore, are very helpful in building visual-motor control as well as directional skills. Remember, however, that the grid map games are only one part of the *A Sense of Direction* activity guide and should not be pulled out to be used in isolation but rather in conjunction with the whole program. Samples of completed grid maps can be found in the appendix beginning on page 209.

You will make floor grids with tape for three-dimensional space activities. Instructions for making floor grids are explained on page 104. Floor grid games incorporate body movement through space and, therefore, are excellent vehicles to learn and apply directional concepts.

You will need to use consistent terminology for grid games. Keep in mind that, although they are interchangeable, the terms *up* and *down* typically refer to two-dimensional flat surfaces while *forward* and *backward* usually refer to three-dimensional spaces. Again, diagonal movement is *not* a component of these activities. When starting a grid game, help the child find the starting square and stay oriented in the same direction throughout the game.

Two-Dimensional Space: Grid Map Games

Follow the Path

Purpose

To differentiate directional concepts in two-dimensional space. To practice visual motor control.

Materials

Reproducible *Follow the Path* grid maps found on pages 62-69, wide-point highlighting marker and a pencil. A sample of a completed *Follow the Path* is included on page 209.

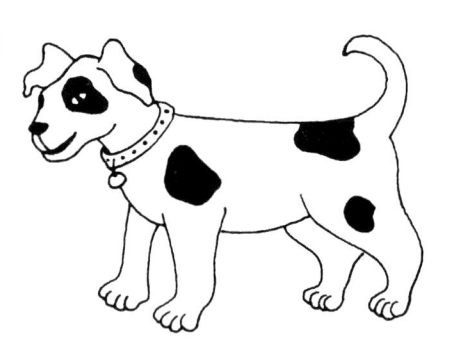

Procedure

- Choose a *Follow the Path* grid map to photocopy. There are eight themes to choose from: Mouse to Cheese, Rocket to Moon, Bee to Flower, Dog to Dog House, Fish to Fishbowl, Bird to Nest, Frog to Lilypad and Child to Bed. In the instructions below, the Mouse to Cheese theme is used as an example.

- Before the game, use the wide-point highlighting marker to draw a path from the start to the finish. Make sure to draw only horizontal and vertical lines. Use the grid lines as guides by tracing over them to draw the path. Now you are ready to start the game.

- Tell the child, "I made a path from the mouse to the cheese. Watch me as I use my finger to follow the path. Listen to me as I tell which way I am going—left, right, up, or down."

- Place your finger on the mouse and trace the highlighted path to the cheese. Say, "left, right, up and down" as you trace.

- Tell the child, "Now you follow the path with your finger. Remember to tell me which way you are going—left, right, up or down."

- After the child has traced the path with his finger, continue instructions by saying, "Now use your pencil to trace the path. Put your pencil on the mouse and draw a line all the way to the cheese. Try to keep your pencil line on the highlighted path. Remember to tell me which way you are going."

Observe

Can the child differentiate directional concepts? Can he project directional concepts onto the paper? Is he able to use directional language concepts accurately to say "left, right, up and down" while tracing?

Observe the child's visual-motor control. Can the child control the pencil well enough to stay on the highlighted line?

More Ideas

Allow the child to use the highlighting marker to draw the path.

Use the blank grid map found on page 204 to make your own *Follow the Path* game. Ask the child to give you ideas for themes.

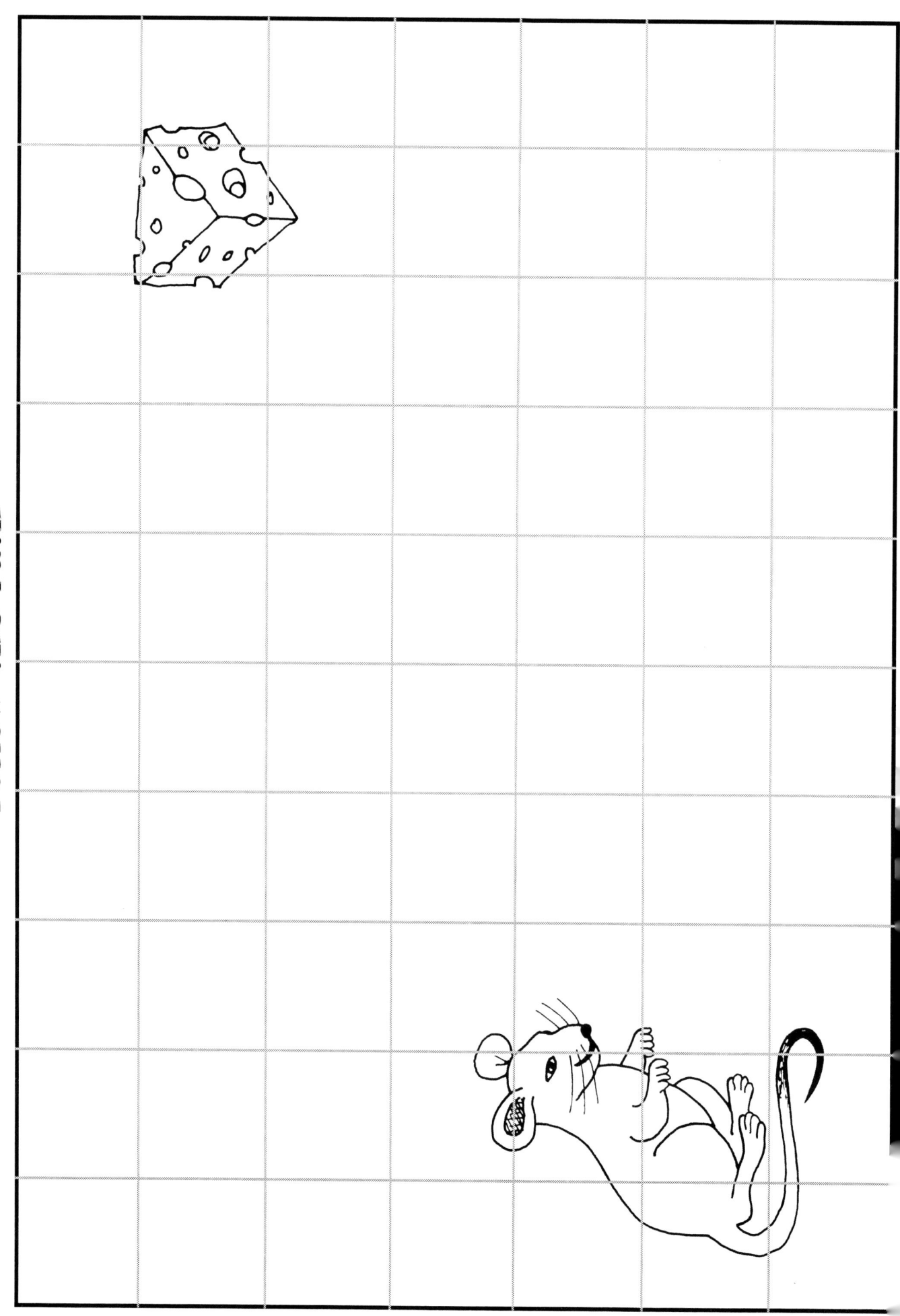

Follow the Path

63

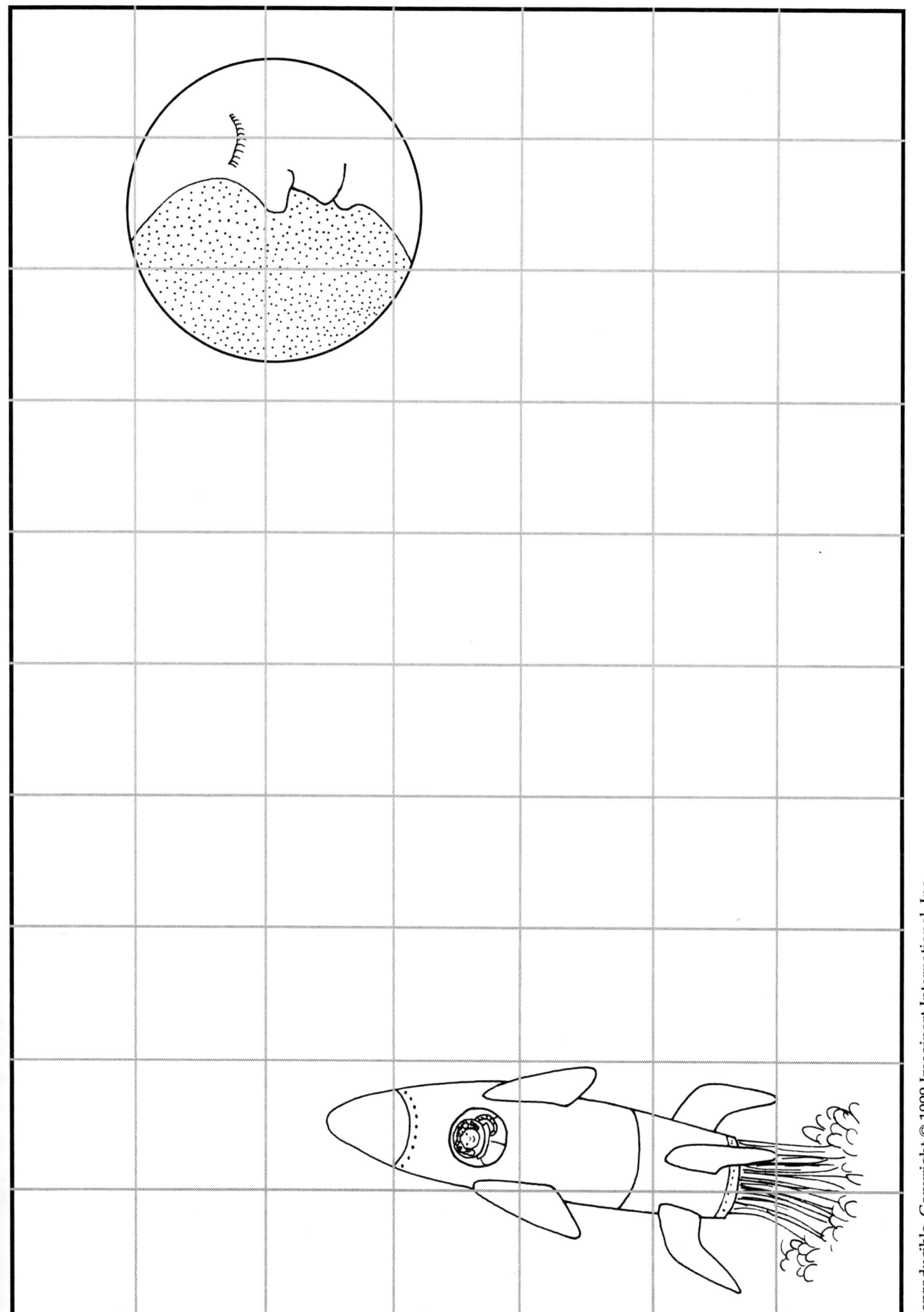

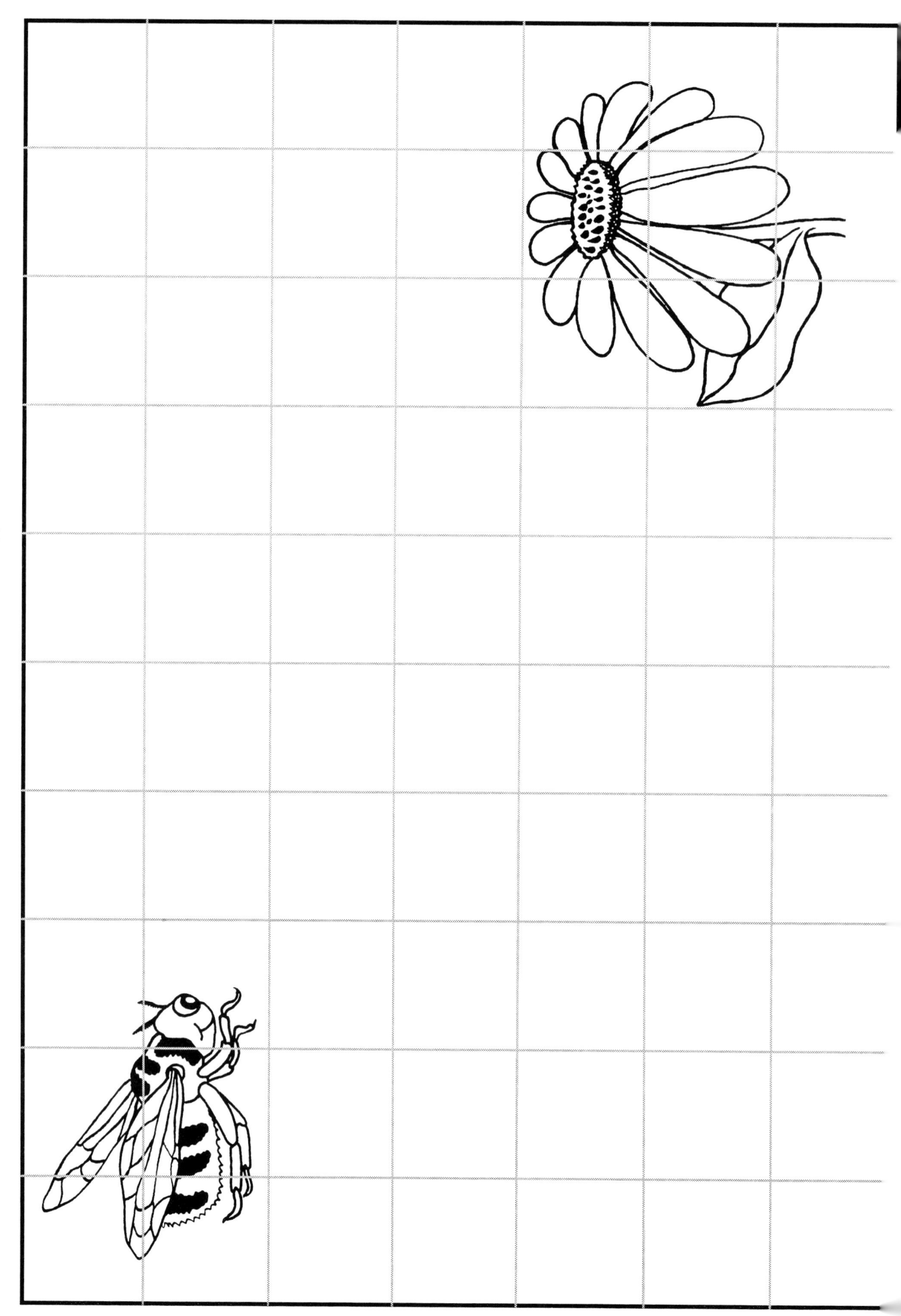

Follow the Path

65

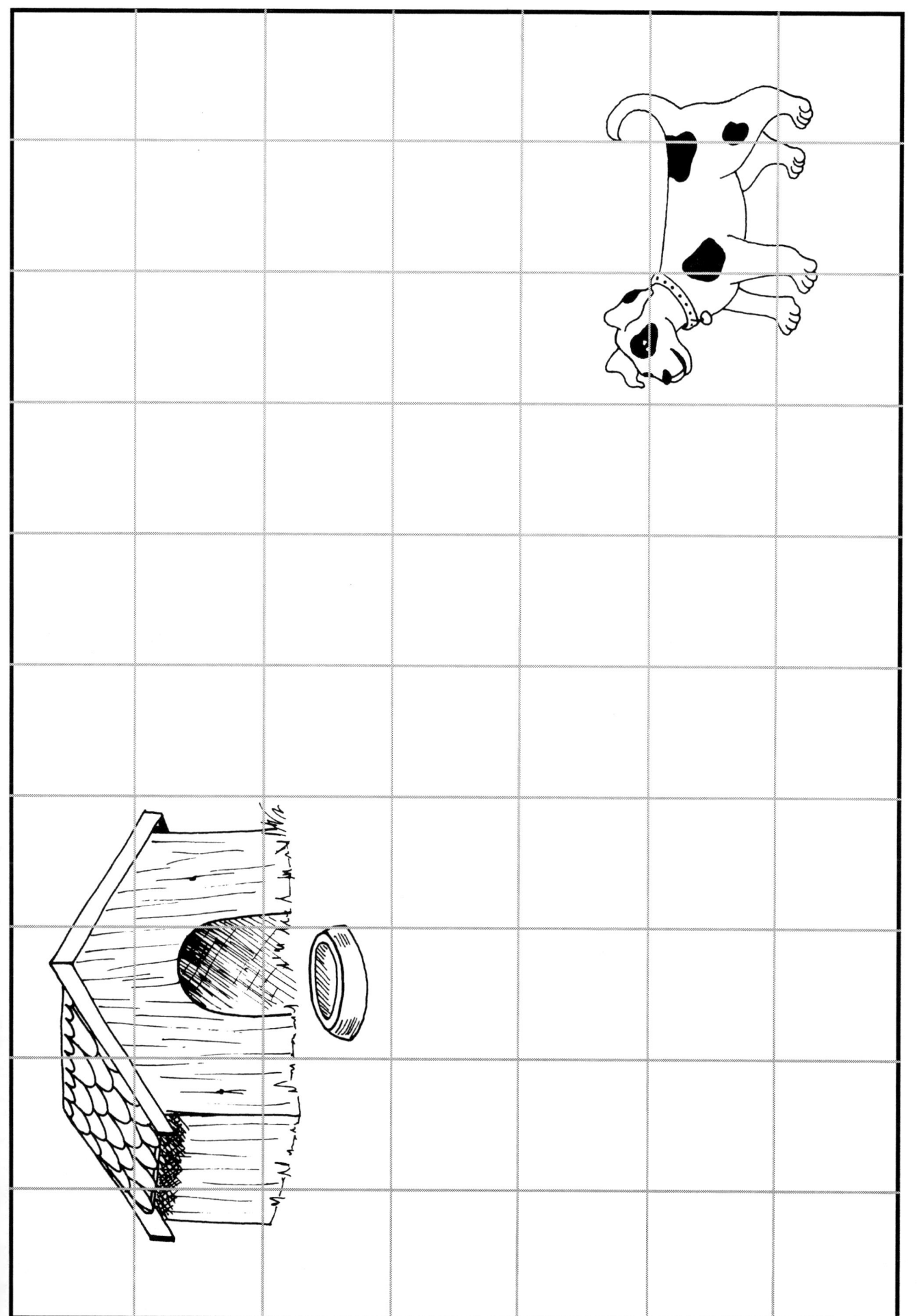

Follow the Path

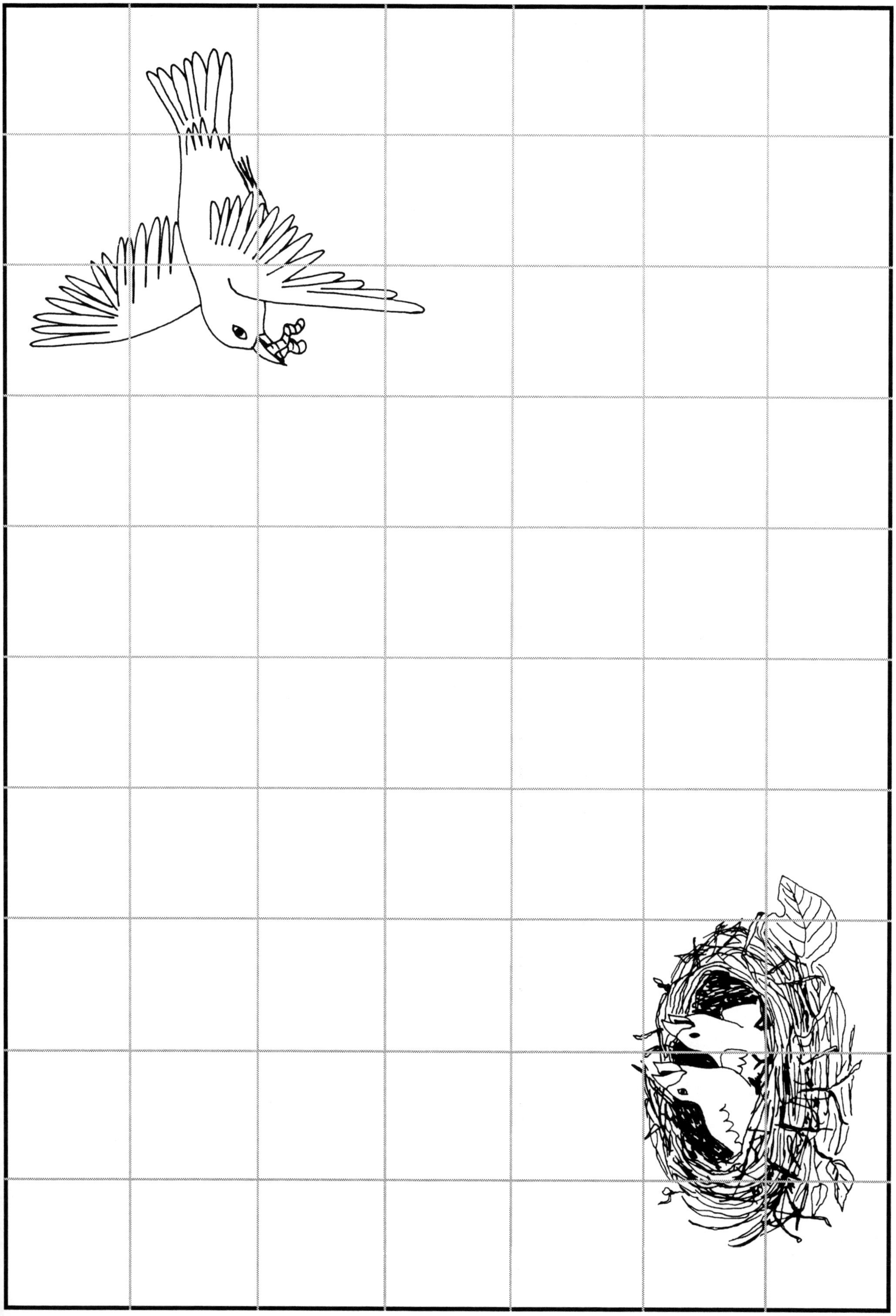

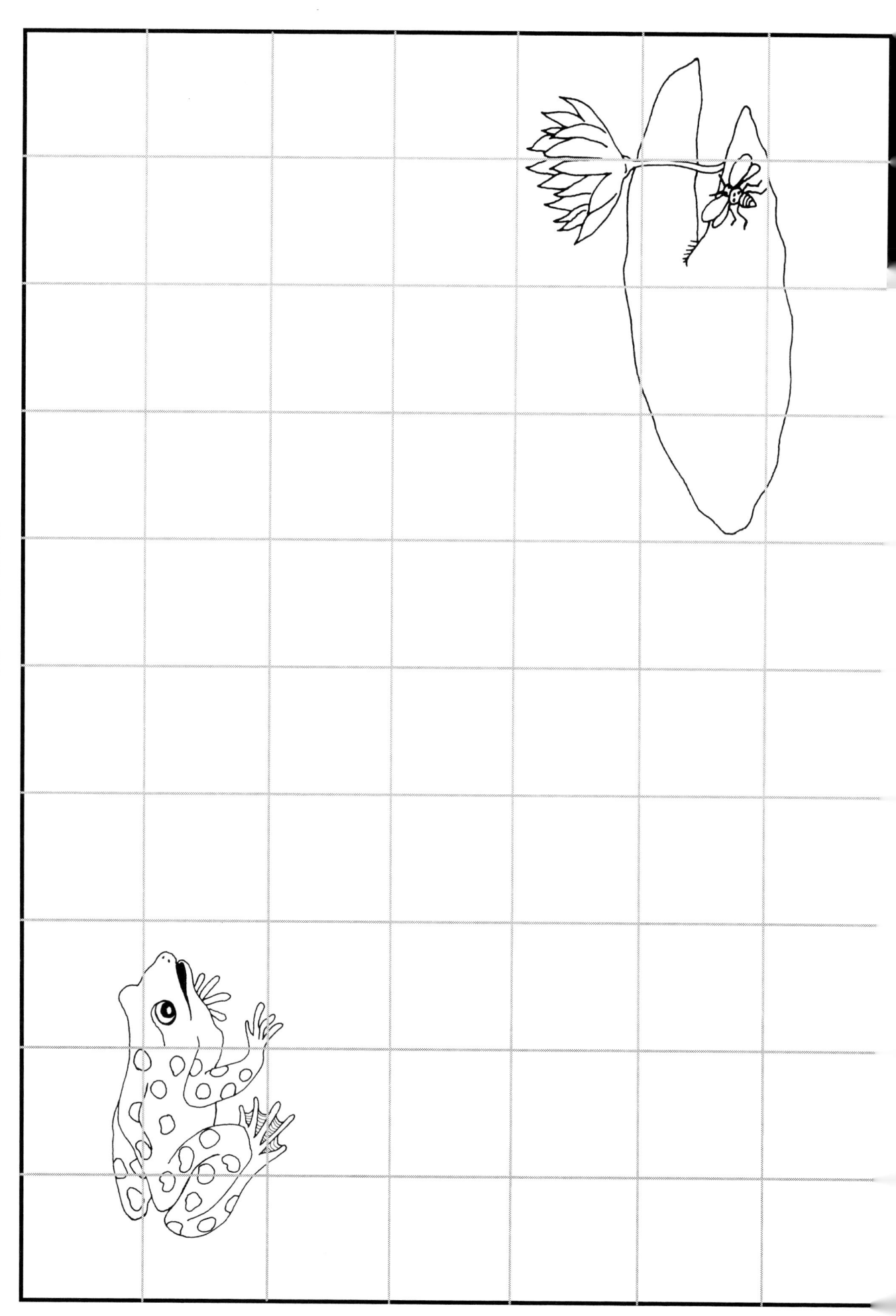

Follow the Path

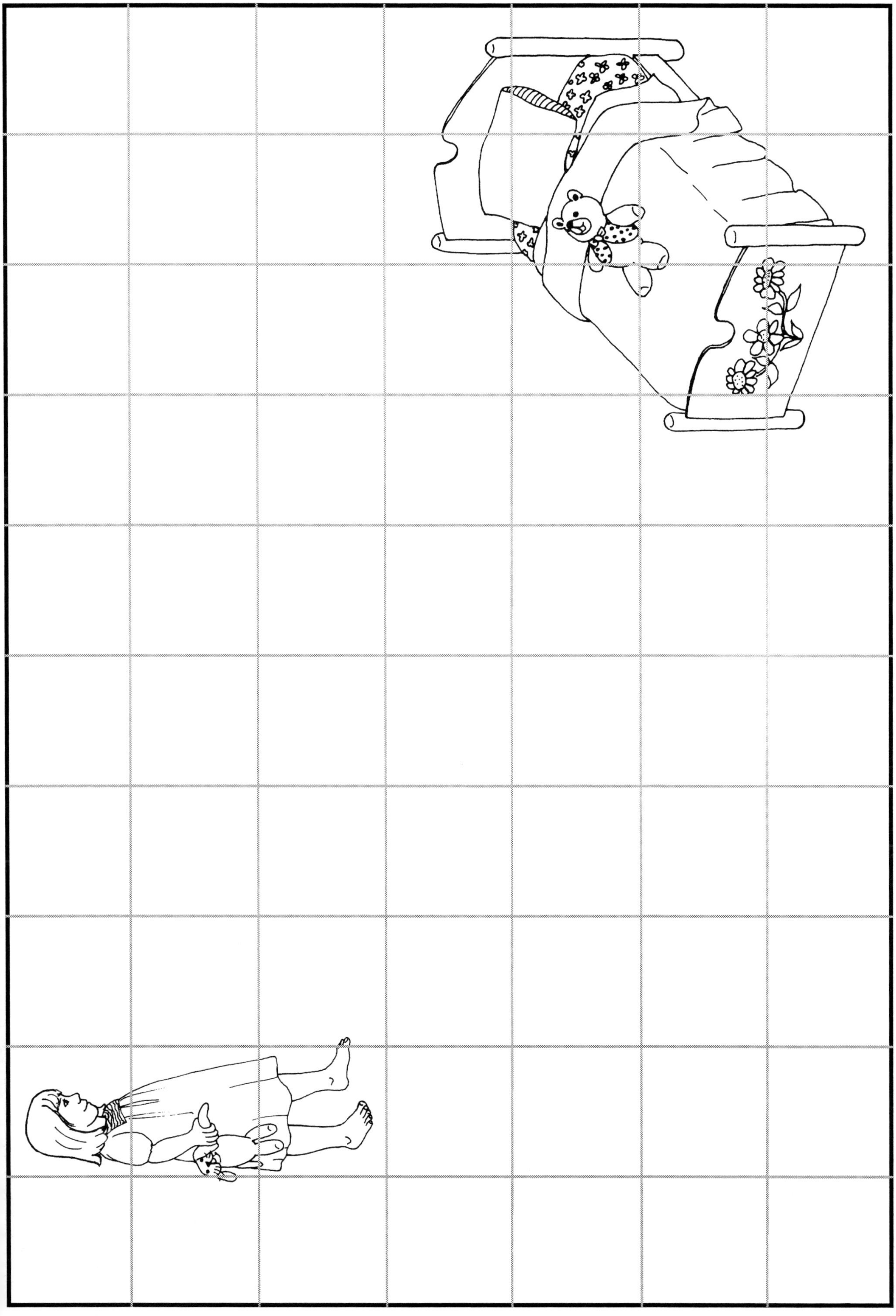

Make a Map

Purpose

To differentiate directional concepts in two-dimensional space. To practice visual motor control.

Materials

Reproducible *Make a Map* grid maps found on pages 72-75, colored pencils, pencil and a sheet of lined paper. A sample of a completed *Make a Map* is included on page 209.

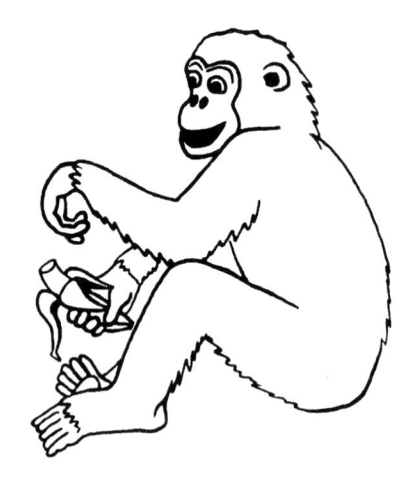

Procedure

- Choose a *Make a Map* grid map to photocopy. There are four themes to choose from: a Carnival, a Grocery Store, a Mall and a Zoo. In the instructions below, the Carnival theme is used as an example.

- Before the game, discuss the Carnival grid map with the child. Say, "Look at all of the places at the carnival that you can go to. Decide where you want to go. Use your pencil and paper to write the names of the places you want to go in the order you want to go to them. Here is an example:

    1) roller coaster

    2) water slide

    3) cotton candy stand"

- Tell the child, "Put your pencil on the starting square. Draw a line to the first place on your list, the roller coaster. Then, draw a line from the roller coaster to the second place on your list, the water slide. Continue until you have drawn a line to each place in order. Remember, you can only go up, down, left or right. When you are finished, put your pencil down."

- Continue instructions by saying, "Now go back to the beginning and put your finger on the starting square. Trace the pencil line with your finger. This time, tell me which way you are going—left, right, up or down."

LEVEL 3—ENVIRONMENT AS A REFERENCE POINT

- Allow the child to color the pictures with the colored pencils when finished.

Observe

Can the child plan a route to each place? Is she able to draw a line to each place in correct sequence? Observe the quality of pencil control. Is the child able to differentiate left, right, up and down? Can she project these directional concepts onto the paper to trace in the correct direction? Is she able to use directional language concepts accurately to say "left, right, up and down" while tracing?

More Ideas

Use a blank grid map, page 205, to create your own *Make a Map* theme. Use this activity to practice and expand related language concepts.

When planning your next field trip, get brochures with real maps before the day of the trip. Spend time discussing where you want to go and planning a route to get there.

Carnival

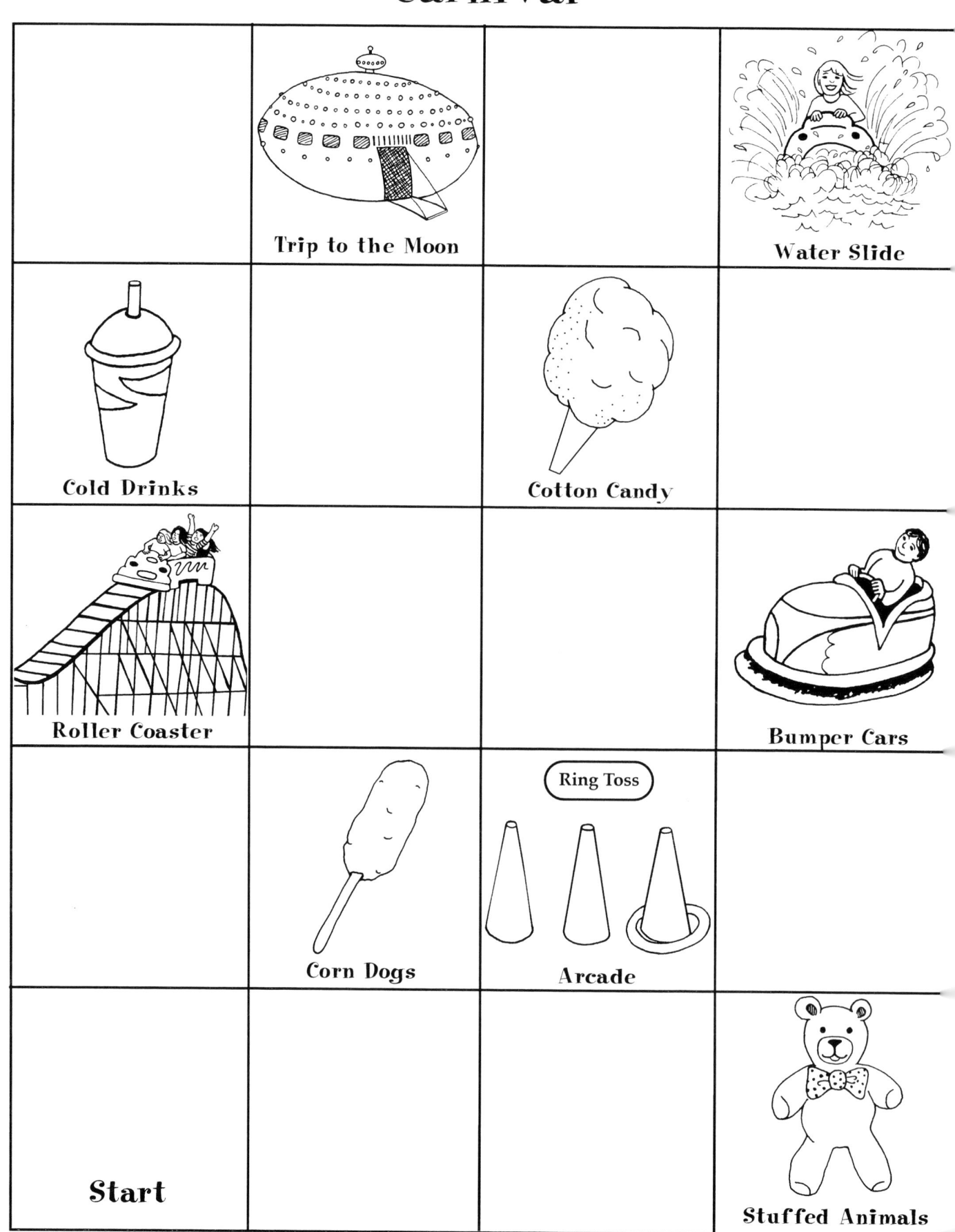

	Trip to the Moon		Water Slide
Cold Drinks		Cotton Candy	
Roller Coaster			Bumper Cars
	Corn Dogs	Ring Toss / Arcade	
Start			Stuffed Animals

Make a Map

Grocery Store

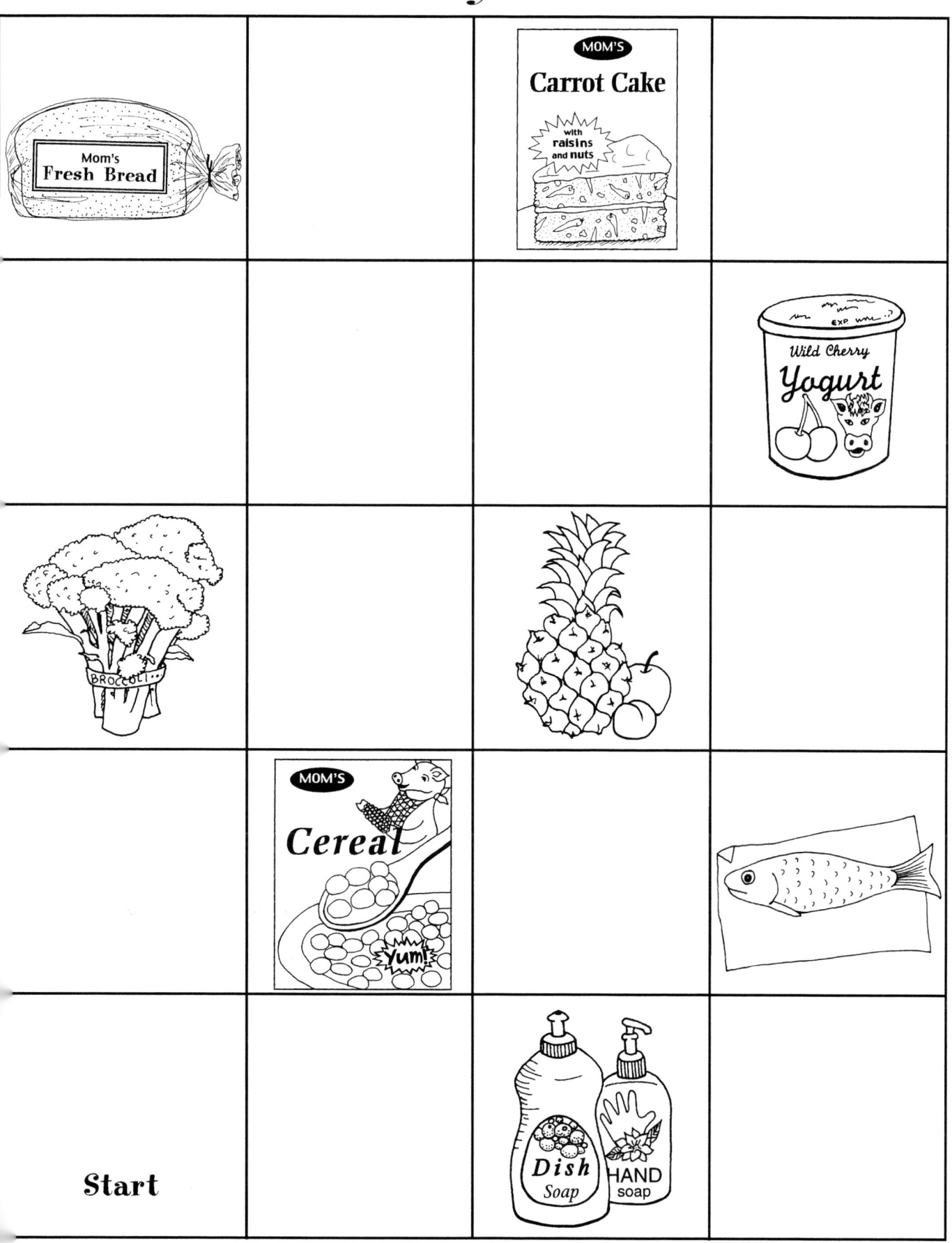

Mom's Fresh Bread		Carrot Cake with raisins and nuts	
			Wild Cherry Yogurt
Broccoli		Pineapple	
	Mom's Cereal Yum!		Fish
Start		Dish Soap / Hand Soap	

Make a Map

Mall

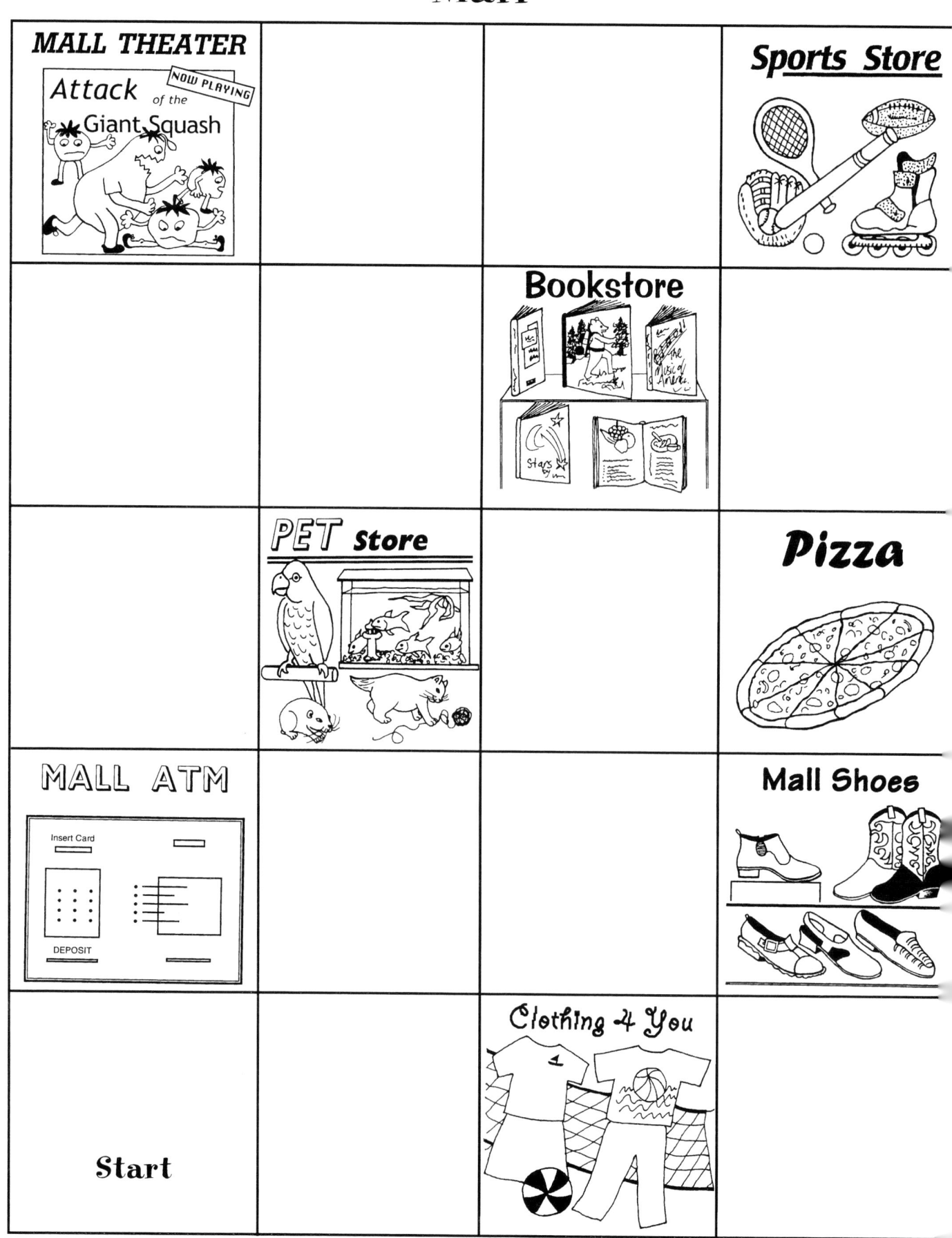

MALL THEATER — Attack of the Giant Squash (NOW PLAYING)			Sports Store
		Bookstore	
	PET Store		Pizza
MALL ATM			Mall Shoes
Start		Clothing 4 You	

Make a Map

Zoo

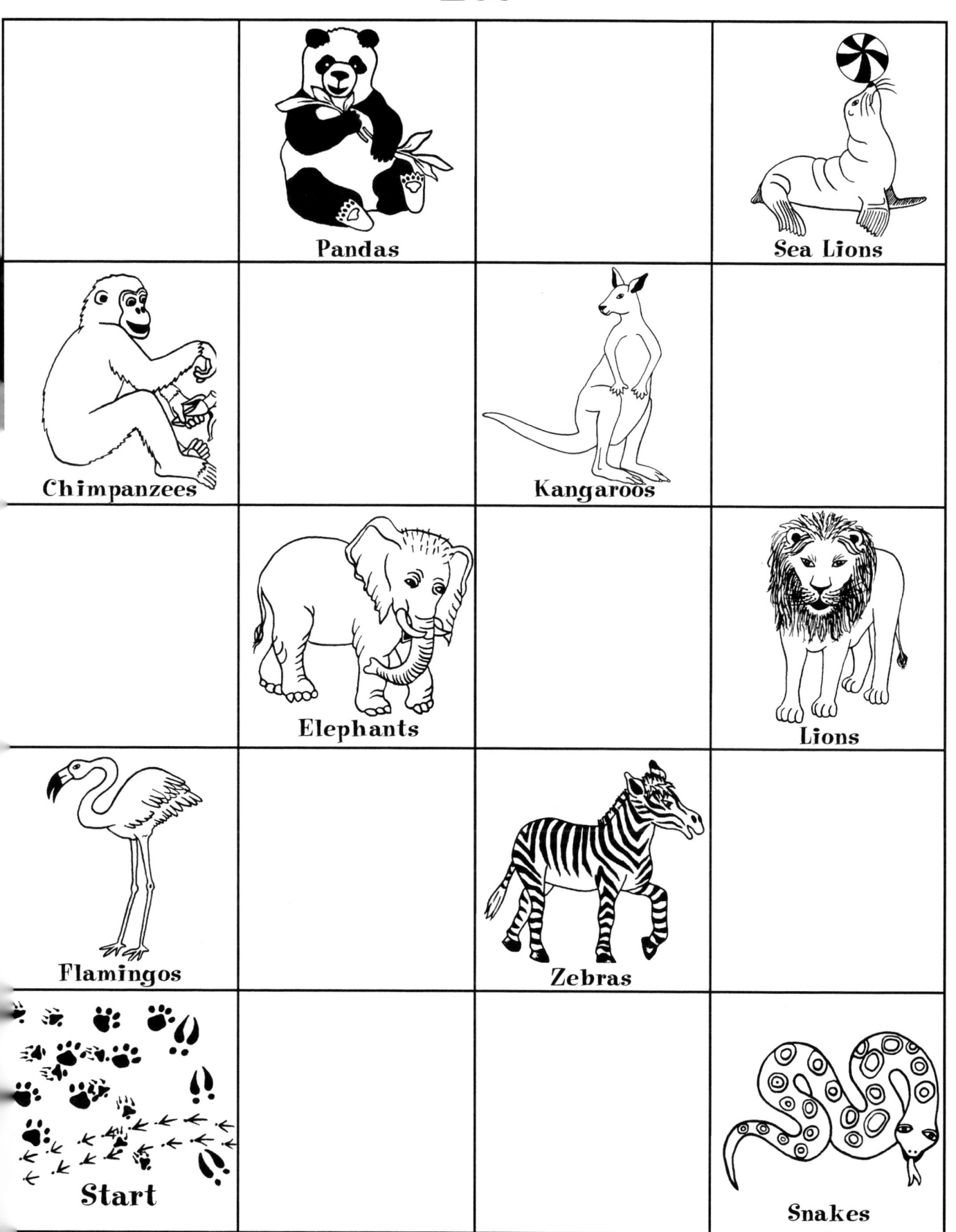

	Pandas		Sea Lions
Chimpanzees		Kangaroos	
	Elephants		Lions
Flamingos		Zebras	
Start			Snakes

Make a Map

Park Your Penny

Purpose

To differentiate directional concepts in two-dimensional space. To follow directional instructions in two-dimensional space. To practice visual-motor control.

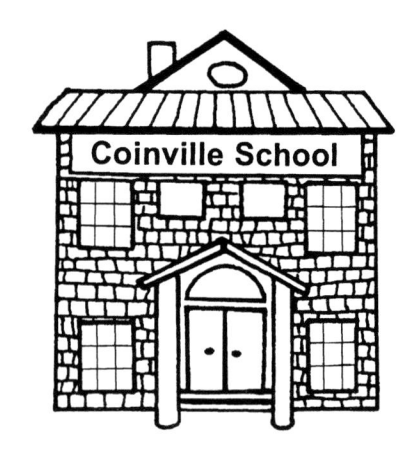

Materials

Map of Coinville, U.S.A. found on page 78 and one penny

Procedure

- Before the game discuss the *Coinville, U.S.A.*, map with the child. Say, "This is a map of a town. Look at the streets, buildings and parking lots. Let's pretend that in *Coinville* people drive pennies instead of cars."

- Tell the child, "Put your penny in the starting circle. Your job is to drive from the starting circle to a parking lot so you can park your penny. There are three parking lots. I will send you to one of them. You have to follow my instructions to get to the correct parking lot. Listen to my left, right, up or down instructions."

- Continue the game by giving directional instructions to one of the parking lots. When the child reaches the correct parking lot, tell him to "park your penny."

- Play again, choosing a different route and different parking lot.

Observe

Can the child differentiate and project directional concepts on to the paper? Is the child able to follow your directional instructions? Observe visual-motor control.

LEVEL 3—ENVIRONMENT AS A REFERENCE POINT

More Ideas

Allow the child to plan the route to a parking lot. Make sure that he verbalizes the correct direction while "driving" the penny.

Use this activity to practice coin recognition, sorting and money skills: Mix pennies, nickels and dimes together on the table. Have the child drive the coins one-by-one to a parking lot. Each coin denomination goes to a separate parking lot. At the end of the game, add up the total value of the coins in each parking lot. Increase the level of difficulty by using coin combinations. For example, tell the child, "We want all the coins in Parking Lot #2 to add up to 45 cents. Drive the correct combination of coins to the parking lot to equal 45 cents."

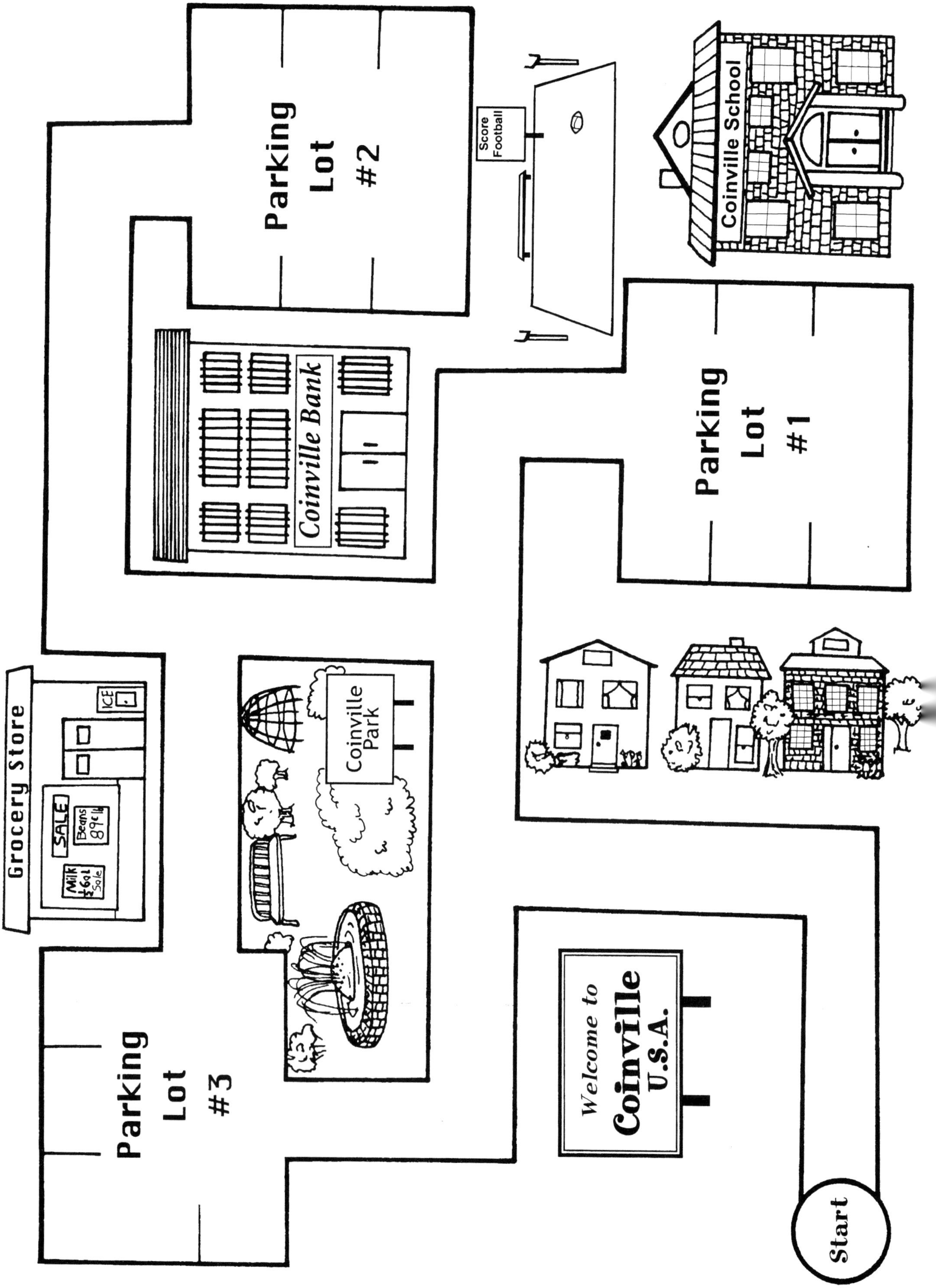
Parking Lot #2
Score Football
Coinville School
Coinville Bank
Parking Lot #1
Grocery Store
SALE
Beans 89¢ lb
Milk $6.01 Sale
ICE
Coinville Park
Parking Lot #3
Welcome to Coinville U.S.A.
Start

Prairie Dog Town

Purpose

To differentiate directional concepts in two-dimensional space. To follow directional instructions. To practice visual-motor control.

Materials

Reproducible *Prairie Dog Town* grid map found on page 81, colored pencils, and a pencil. A sample of a completed *Prairie Dog Town* is included on page 210.

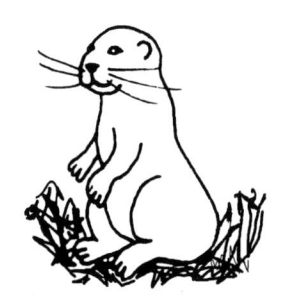

Procedure

- Before the game, discuss the *Prairie Dog* grid map with the child. Talk about the habitats of prairie dogs. Say, "This is a map of an underground prairie dog town. Prairie dogs dig holes, tunnels and rooms underground. They live underground to have shelter from storms and predators. They use some of the underground rooms to store grass and weeds to eat. They sleep in some of the rooms. Other rooms are just for the newborn baby prairie dogs. On warm days prairie dogs leave their underground home and play up on the surface. Sometimes, other animals live nearby in underground homes. Prairie dogs might have snakes or burrowing owls for neighbors."

- Tell the child, "Let's make up a story about a prairie dog. During the story, I will tell you to draw lines. Listen to my left, right, up and down directions carefully—don't end up in the snake hole by mistake!"

- Continue the game by giving directional instructions to the various underground locations. Give instructions in story form as in the following example:

    "It is time for the baby prairie dogs to eat. The mother prairie dog must feed her babies in the nursery. Find the mother prairie dog in her underground room and put your pencil there. Draw a line from the mother to the nursery. Go up one square, go right one square, go up one square, go left one

LEVEL 3—ENVIRONMENT AS A REFERENCE POINT

square. Did you get to the nursery? Now the baby prairie dogs can eat!" When the story is finished, tell the child, "Put your pencil down."

- Continue instructions by saying: "Now you try to remember the story about the prairie dog and tell it to me. As you tell the story, show me where the prairie dog goes by tracing over the pencil line with your finger. Don't forget to use left, right, up and down words."

- When the game is over, allow the child to color the prairie dog town with colored pencils.

Observe

Can the child differentiate and project directional concepts onto the paper? Is she able to follow your directional instructions? Can she retell the story using the correct directional language concepts? Observe pencil control.

More Ideas

Allow the child to make up a prairie dog story and direct you to each location.

Use this activity as part of a science unit on animal habitats.

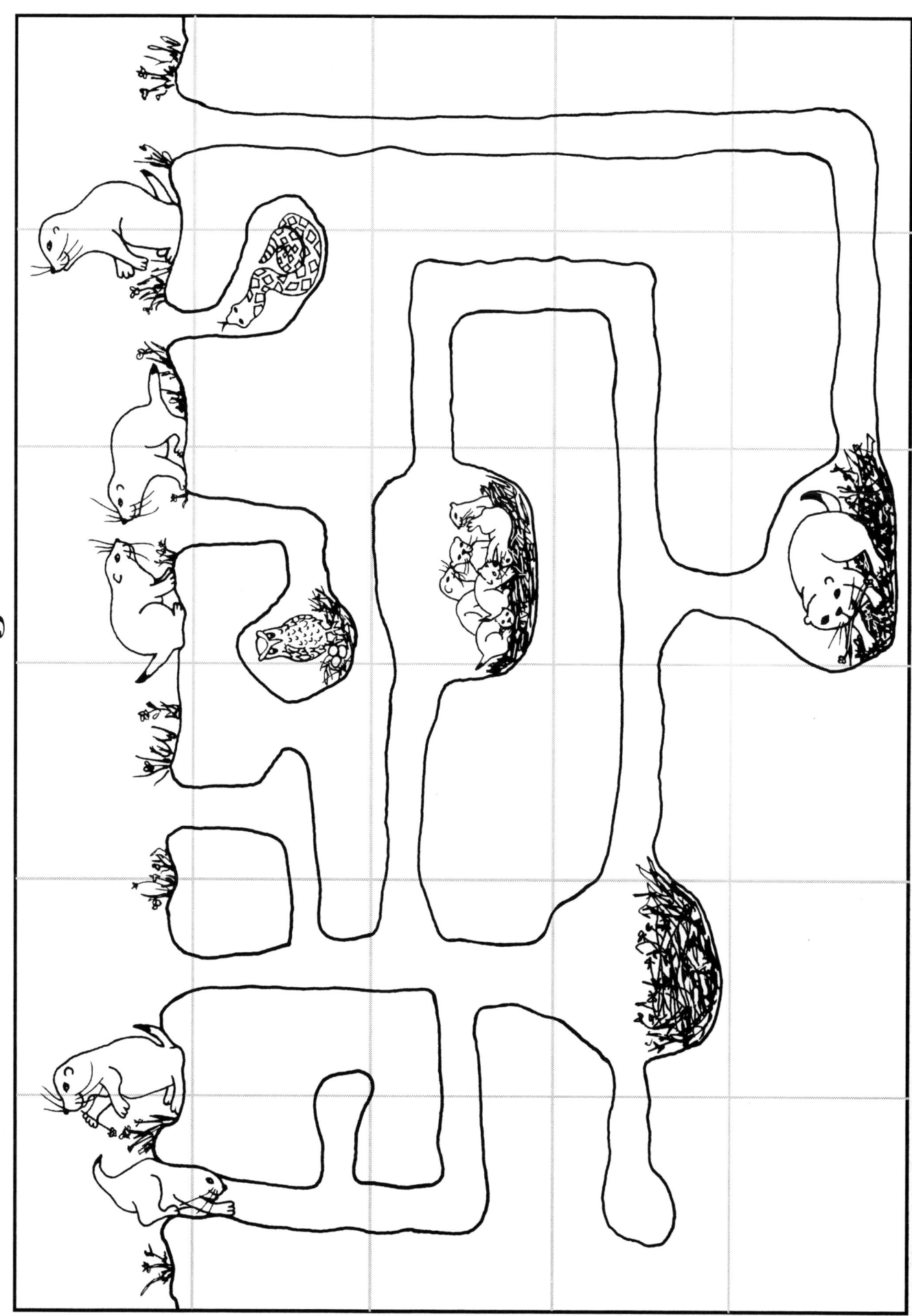

Prairie Dog Town

Animal Parade

Purpose

To differentiate directional concepts in two-dimensional space. To practice numerical sequencing. To practice visual-motor control.

Materials

Reproducible *Animal Parade* grid map found on page 84, pencil and colored pencils. A sample of a completed *Animal Parade* is included on page 210.

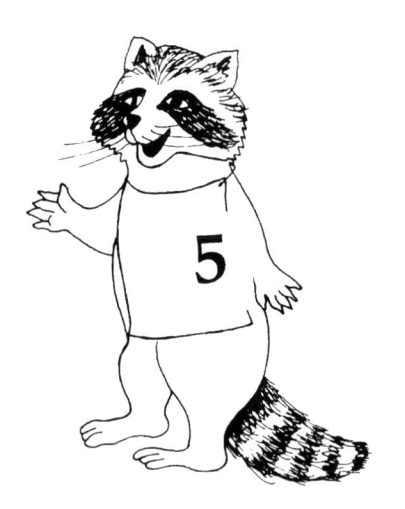

Procedure

- Before the game, print a number in the center of each animal in random order. Now you are ready to begin the game.

- Tell the child, "These animals are going to march in a parade. Each animal has a number. Your job is to find the animals in correct number order so they can march in the parade."

- Continue instructions by saying, "Put your pencil on the starting square. Draw a line to animal number 1. Then, draw a line from animal number 1 to animal number 2. Continue until you have drawn a line to each animal in order. Remember, you can only draw lines that go left, right, up or down. When you are finished, put your pencil down."

- Tell the child, "Now go back to the beginning and put your finger on the starting square. Trace the pencil line with your finger. This time, tell me which way you are going—left, right, up or down."

- Allow the child to decorate the animals with the colored pencils when finished.

Observe

Does the child understand numerical sequencing? Can the child draw a line to each animal in correct order? Observe the quality of pencil con-

LEVEL 3—ENVIRONMENT AS A REFERENCE POINTT

trol. Is the child able to differentiate left, right, up and down? Can the child project these directional concepts onto the paper to trace in the correct direction? Is the child able to use the directional language concepts accurately to say "left, right, up and down" while tracing?

More Ideas

Vary the activity by allowing the child to print numbers in the animals at the beginning of the game.

Combine this activity with a math unit on numerical sequencing.

Save the completed *Animal Parade* grid map to play the floor grid version of this game—*Animal Parade Floor Grid Game,* found on page 120.

Animal Parade

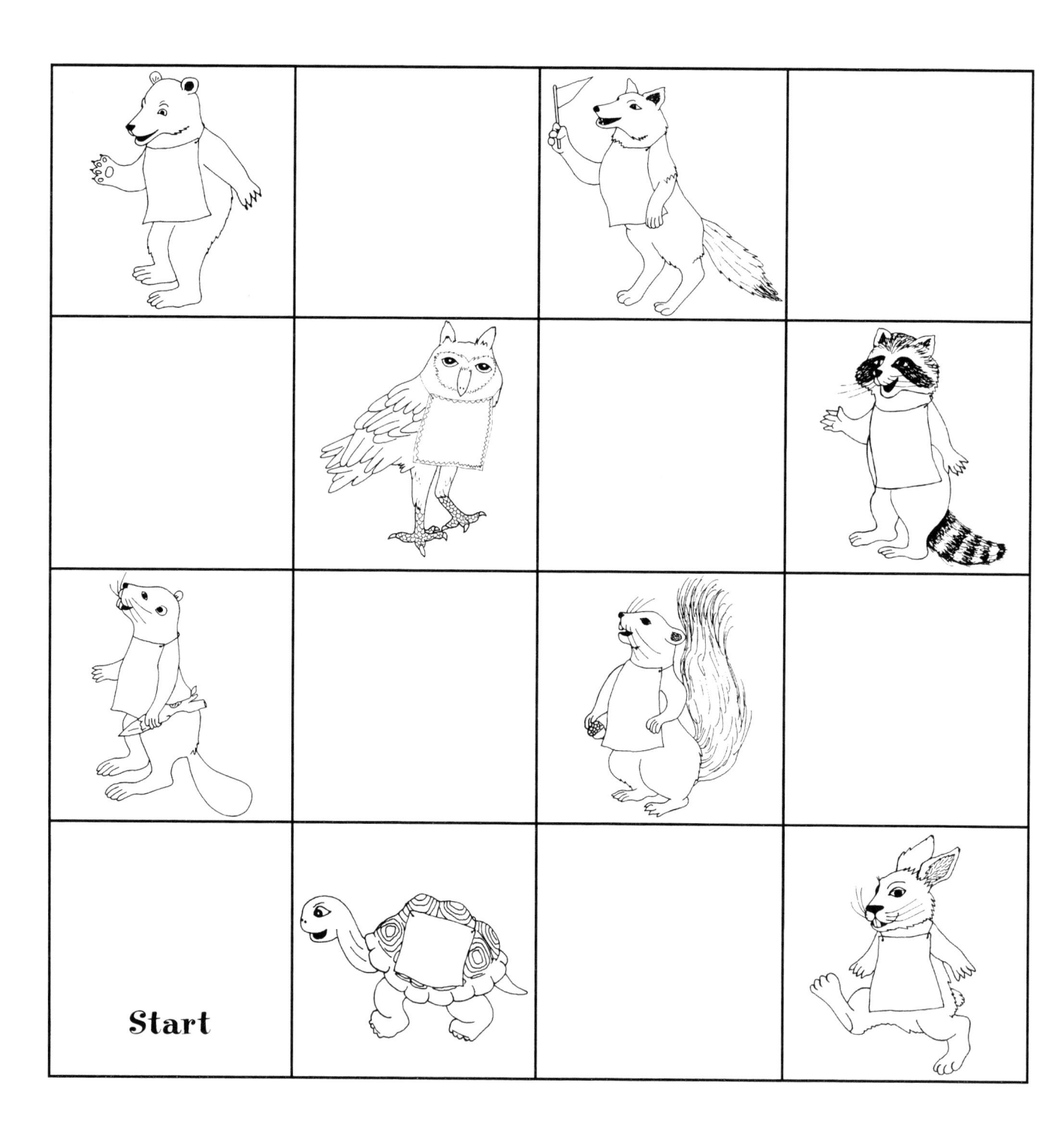

Start

Mixed-Up Socks

Purpose

To differentiate directional concepts in two-dimensional space. To develop visual discrimination and matching skills. To practice visual-motor control.

Materials

Reproducible *Mixed-Up Socks* grid map found on page 87, pencil and colored pencils. A sample of a completed *Mixed-Up Socks* is included on page 211.

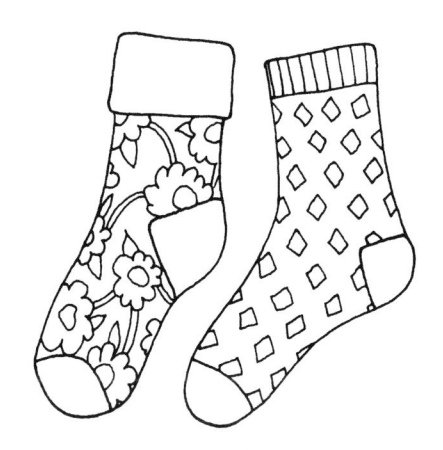

Procedure

- Tell the child, "These socks are all mixed up. Your job is to put the socks that look the same into matching pairs."

- Continue instructing the child by saying, "Put your pencil in the starting square. Draw a line to a sock. You can go to any sock you choose. Then, find the sock that matches it and draw a line to it. Continue until you have drawn a line to each sock and its match. Remember, you can only draw lines that go left, right, up or down. When you are finished, put your pencil down."

- Tell the child, "Now go back to the beginning and put your finger on the starting square. Trace the pencil line with your finger. This time, tell me which way you are going—left, right, up or down."

- Allow the child to decorate the socks with the colored pencils when finished.

Observe

Can the child discriminate the visual similarities and differences among the socks? Does the child understand the concept of matching? Observe the quality of pencil control. Is the child able to differentiate left, right, up and down? Can the child project these directional concepts onto the paper to trace the correct direction? Is the child able to use the directional language concepts accurately to say "left, right, up and down" while tracing?

More Ideas

Use real socks of various colors, sizes, patterns and styles to build visual discrimination and matching skills. Encourage the child to describe the similarities and differences among the socks. Practice rolling each matching pair of socks into a ball to develop dexterity. Then, allow the child to throw the sock balls into a laundry basket to practice visual-motor coordination.

Save the completed *Mixed-Up Socks* grid map to play the floor grid version of this game—*Mixed-Up Socks Floor Grid Game* found on page 126.

Mixed-Up Socks

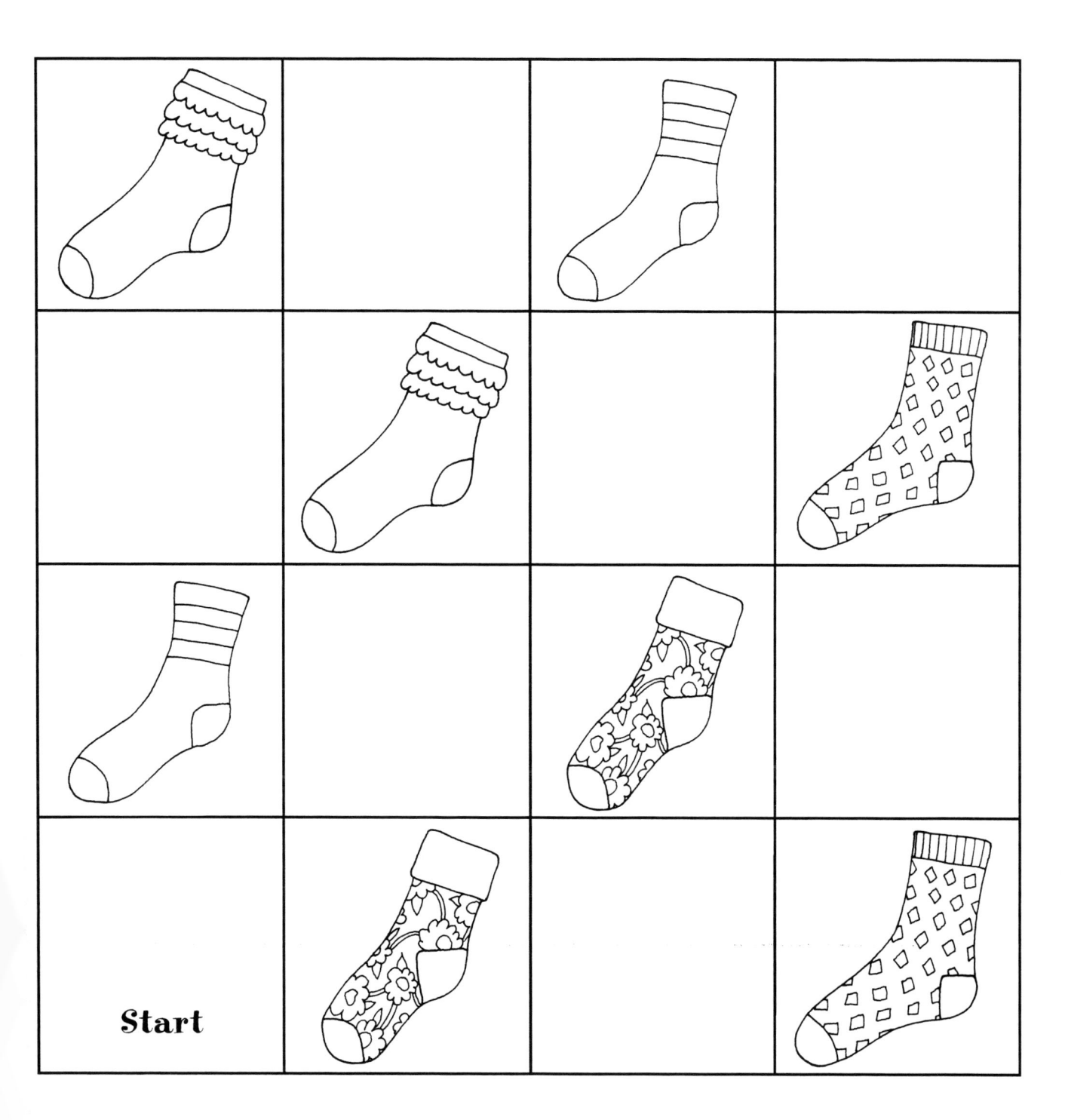

Start			

Mail Delivery

Purpose

To differentiate directional concepts in two-dimensional space. To practice sequencing in alphabetical order. To practice visual-motor control.

Materials

Reproducible *Mail Delivery* grid map found on page 90, pencil and colored pencils

Procedure

- Before the game, print a name on the line on each envelope in random order. The names can be classmates, family members or friends. The first time you play, simplify the game by printing only three names on three envelopes. This will make sequencing in alphabetical order easier for beginners. Now you are ready to start the game.

- Tell the child, "These envelopes are for your friends (or classmates or family). Your first job is to find each name in alphabetical order. There are numbered lines at the bottom of the page. Print each name in alphabetical order on the numbered lines."

- After the child has sequenced the names alphabetically, continue the instructions by saying, "Put your pencil in the starting square. Draw a line to the envelope with the first name. Then, draw a line from the envelope with the first name to the envelope with the second name. Continue until you have drawn a line to all the names in alphabetical order. Use your numbered list to help you. Remember, you can only draw lines that go left, right, up or down. When you are finished, put your pencil down."

- Tell the child, "Now go back to the beginning and put your finger on the starting square. Trace the pencil line with your finger. This time, tell me which way you are going—left, right, up or down."

- Allow the child to decorate the envelopes with the colored pencils.

LEVEL 3—ENVIRONMENT AS A REFERENCE POINT

Observe

Does the child understand alphabetical order? Can he draw a line to each envelope in the correct sequence? Observe the quality of pencil control. Is he able to differentiate left, right, up and down? Can the child project these directional concepts onto the paper to trace in the correct direction? Is the child able to use directional language concepts accurately to say "left, right, up and down" while tracing?

More Ideas

Include this activity with a unit on alphabetizing.

Expand this activity by using real envelopes to practice writing addresses. Help the child to memorize his home address.

Encourage the child to make a greeting card or write a letter to enclose in the envelope.

Invite a mail carrier to the classroom or plan a field trip to the post office.

Save the completed *Mail Delivery* grid map to play the floor grid version of this game—*Mail Delivery Floor Grid Game* found on page 132.

Mail Delivery

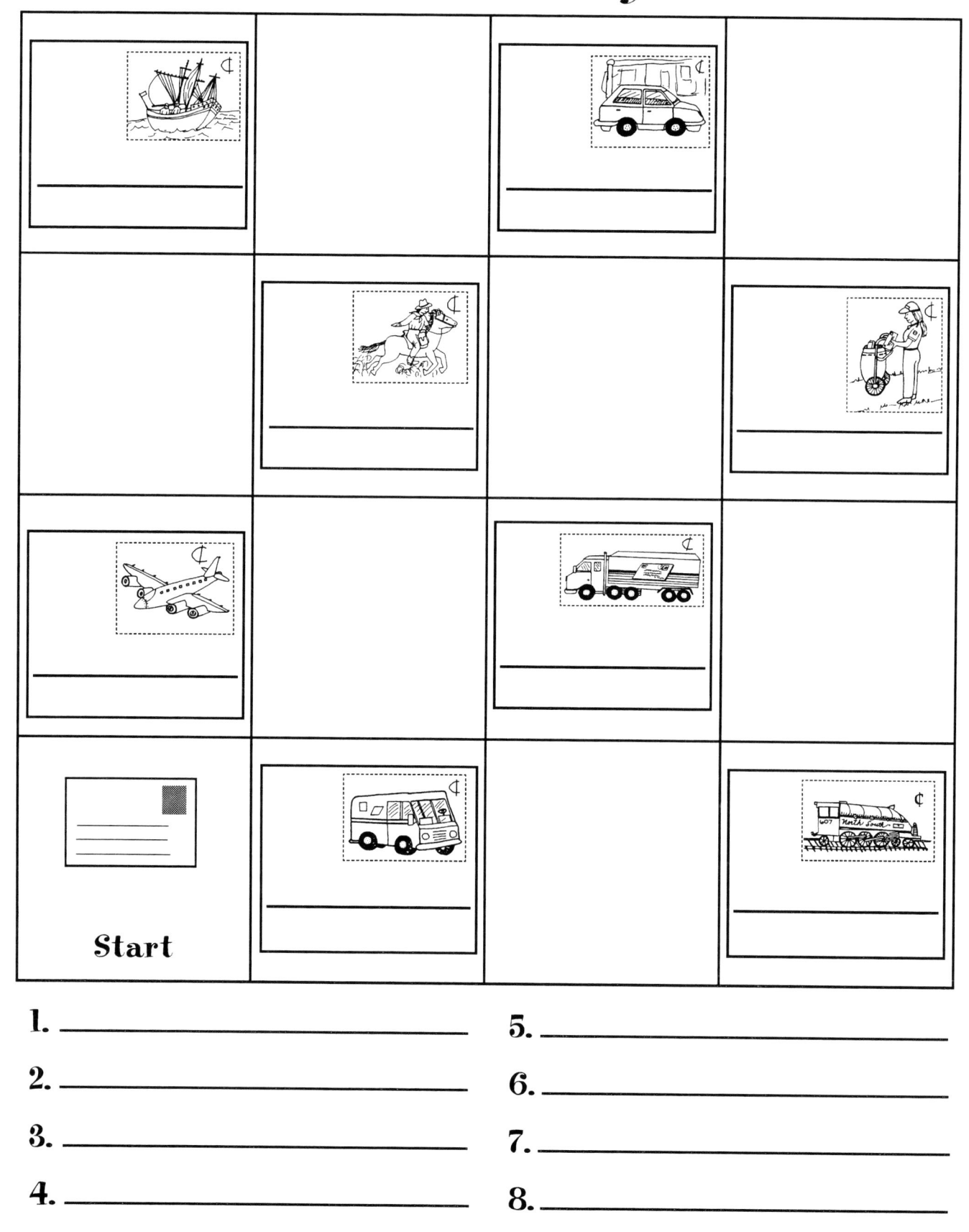

1. _____
2. _____
3. _____
4. _____

5. _____
6. _____
7. _____
8. _____

Reproducible. Copyright © 1999 Imaginart International, Inc.

Secret Word

Purpose

To differentiate directional concepts in two-dimensional space. To follow directional instructions. To practice visual-motor control. To practice reading and spelling skills.

Materials

Blank *Secret Word* grid map on page 93 and a pencil. A sample of a completed *Secret Word* is included on page 211.

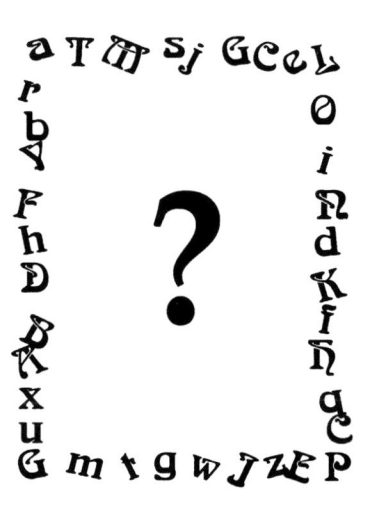

Procedure

- Before starting the game, choose a simple spelling word or vocabulary word (at the child's reading level) to be the "secret word." Using the blank grid map and pencil, print each letter of the secret word in a grid square. Mix the letters so that they are in random order. Now you are ready to start the game.

- Tell the child, "There is a secret word hidden in these squares. Your job is to unscramble the letters to spell the secret word."

- Continue instructing the child by saying, "Put your pencil on the starting square. I will give you instructions to draw a line from the starting square to each letter of the secret word. I will tell you to go right, left, up or down. For example, I may say, 'Go up one square, go right two squares.' When you get to a square with a letter inside, print the letter on the line below.

- Tell the child, "When you print all of the letters in the correct order, try to guess the secret word."

Observe

Does the child move the pencil quickly and automatically in response to your right, left, up and down instructions? Can the child print each letter on the line and then return to the correct grid square without confusion?

LEVEL 3—ENVIRONMENT AS A REFERENCE POINT

Observe the quality of pencil control.

More Ideas

Combine this activity with a language arts unit.

Expand this activity by asking the student to define the secret word and use it in a sentence, spell the secret word from memory with her eyes closed and write the secret word in cursive.

Allow the child to choose the secret word, print it in the grid squares and direct you to each letter in correct order.

Play the floor grid version of this game—*Secret Word Floor Grid Game* found on page 138.

Secret Word

Start			

Reproducible. Copyright © 1999 Imaginart International, Inc.

Three-Ways Maze

Purpose

To differentiate directional concepts in two-dimensional space. To practice giving and following directional instructions in two-dimensional space. To practice visual perception and visual-motor skills.

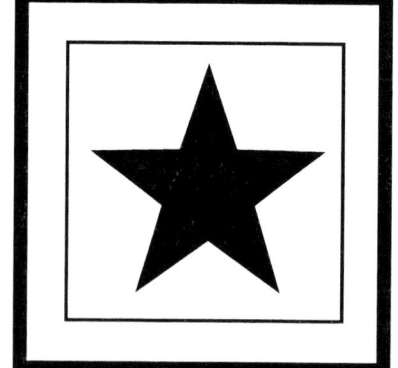

Materials

Reproducible *Three-Ways Maze* grid map found on page 96, and pink, blue and yellow highlighting markers. A sample of a completed *Three-Ways Maze* is included on page 212.

Procedure

- Photocopy the *Three-Ways Maze* grid map.

- Tell the child, "This maze has many different paths. All the paths lead to the star. Your job is to find three different ways to get to the star."

- Continue instructing the child by saying, "Use the pink marker to make the first path. Put the marker on Start #1 and trace over a path. You can go any way you want, but you must tell me which direction you are going by saying 'up, down, left, or right'."

- When the child reaches the star, say, "Now use the blue marker to trace a new path. Begin the blue path at Start #2. Try to avoid all of the pink paths. Remember to tell me which way you are going."

- When the child reaches the star, continue by saying, "Next, use the yellow marker to trace one more new path. Begin the yellow path at Start #3. This time try to avoid both the pink and blue paths to reach the star. Can you find a new way? Remember to tell me which way you are going."

LEVEL 3—ENVIRONMENT AS A REFERENCE POINT

Observe

Can the child use accurate directional language to describe the route? Consider the child's visual-perceptual and visual-motor skills. Is she able to find three different paths? Can the child trace over the path with smooth line control? Are the corners squared or rounded?

More Ideas

Use a blank grid map, page 207, to make your own *Three-Ways Maze*.

Allow the child to make her own *Three-Ways Maze*.

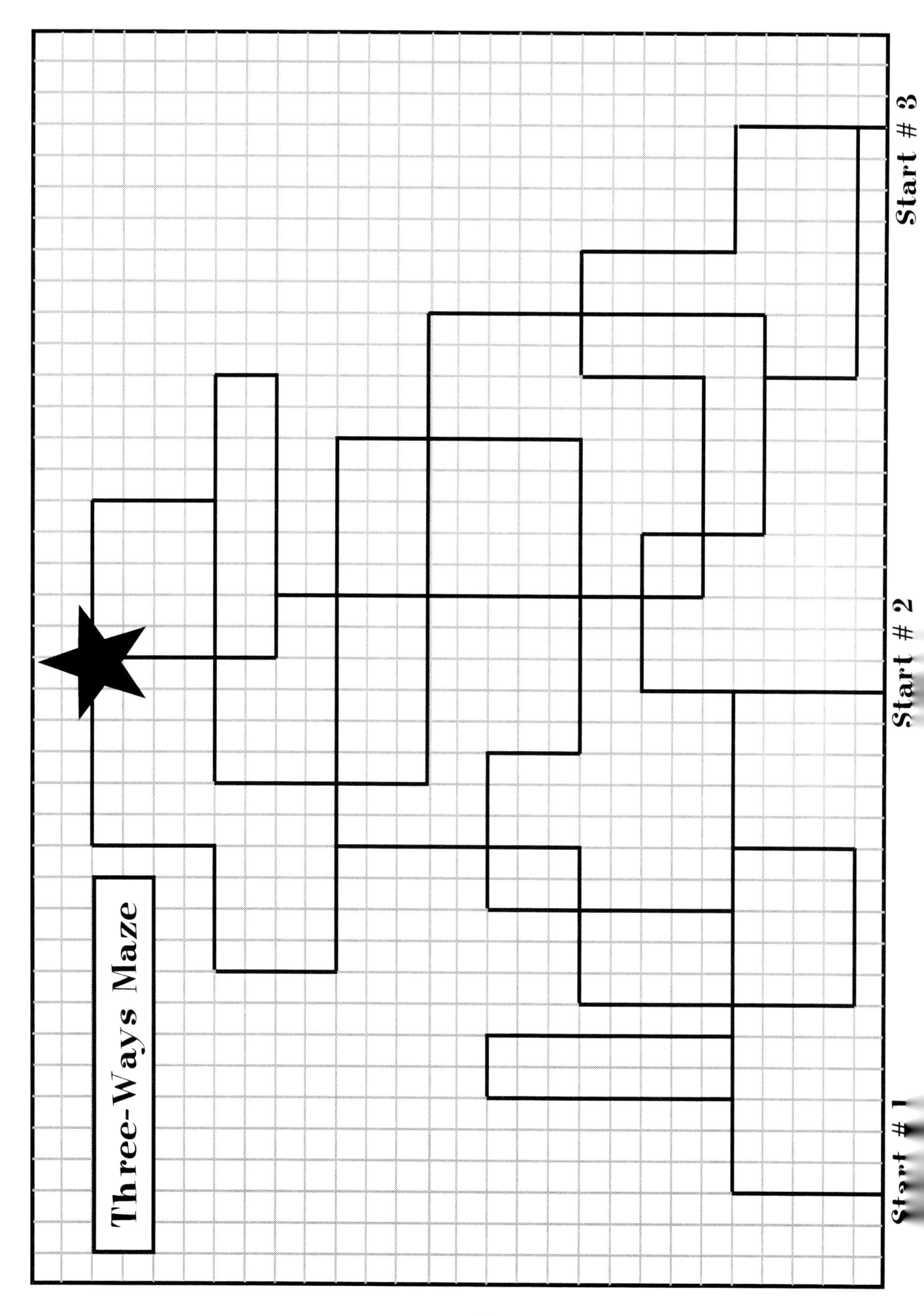

Three-Ways Maze

Start #1

Start #2

Start #3

Secret Door

Purpose

To differentiate directional concepts in two-dimensional space. To practice giving and following directional instructions in two-dimensional space. To practice visual perception and visual-motor skills.

Materials

Reproducible *Secret Door* grid map on page 99, highlighting marker, small Post-it Notes (1 1/2" x 2"), small stickers and a pencil. A sample of a completed *Secret Door* is included on page 212.

Procedure

- Photocopy the *Secret Door* grid map.

- Before the game, place a Post-it Note in the three spaces provided. Position each Post-it Note like a door that can open. Draw a doorknob and a question mark on each Post-it Note. Hide a small sticker behind one of the Post-it Note doors.

- Tell the child, "This game is called *Secret Door*. There is a sticker hidden behind one of these little doors. Which door do you think is the Secret Door?"

- Continue instructing the child by saying, "Put your marker on 'start' and trace a path to one of the doors. You can follow any path you like but you must tell me which direction you are going—up, down, left, or right."

- Tell the child, "When you get to a door, you may open it. If the sticker is behind the door, you win. If the sticker is not behind the door, you must go back to 'start' and try again until you find the secret door."

LEVEL 3—ENVIRONMENT AS A REFERENCE POINT

Observe

Can the child use accurate directional language to describe the route?
Can the child trace over the path with smooth line control?

More Ideas

Use a blank grid map, page 208, to make your own *Secret Door* maze.

Allow the child to make his own *Secret Door* maze.

Secret Door

Start

File Cabinet

Purpose

To differentiate directional concepts in two-dimensional space. To practice giving and following directional instructions in two-dimensional space. To practice visual memory and sequencing.

Materials

Reproducible *File Cabinet* grid map on page 102, fifteen small Post-it Notes (1 1/2"x 2"), small stickers and a pencil

Procedure

- Photocopy the *File Cabinet* grid map.

- Before the game, hold the sheet vertically and place one Post-it Note in each space provided to create little "drawers." Draw a small line on each Post-it Note to represent a handle. Hide one small sticker behind the Post-it Note in the first row, last drawer on the right. Now you are ready to begin the game.

- Tell the child, "Pretend that each little piece of paper is a drawer in a tiny file cabinet. I have hidden a sticker in one of the drawers. Follow my instructions to find which drawer the sticker is in."

- Continue instructing the child by saying, "Look in the first row and open the last drawer on the right. Is a sticker there? Remember *what* it is and *where* it is."

- Tell the child, "Now I will hide another sticker in a different drawer. I will give you instructions to find it. When you find it, remember *what* it is and *where* it is."

- Repeat the sequence until there are three stickers hidden in different drawers.

- Continue the game by saying, "Now it is your turn to tell me where the

---

LEVEL 3—ENVIRONMENT AS A REFERENCE POINT

stickers are hiding. You must remember where all three stickers are hiding. Give me instructions to find each sticker in order. Use specific direction words when you give me instructions, like this:

> 5th row, last drawer on the right
>
> 3rd row, middle drawer
>
> 2nd row, first drawer on the left"

Observe

Can the child follow your instructions accurately? When the child gives you instructions, does she use directional language concepts accurately? Assess visual memory and sequencing. Is the child able to recall the sticker and its location in correct order?

More Ideas

Make the game more challenging by increasing the number of stickers in the sequence.

Allow the child to hide the stickers for you.

File Cabinet

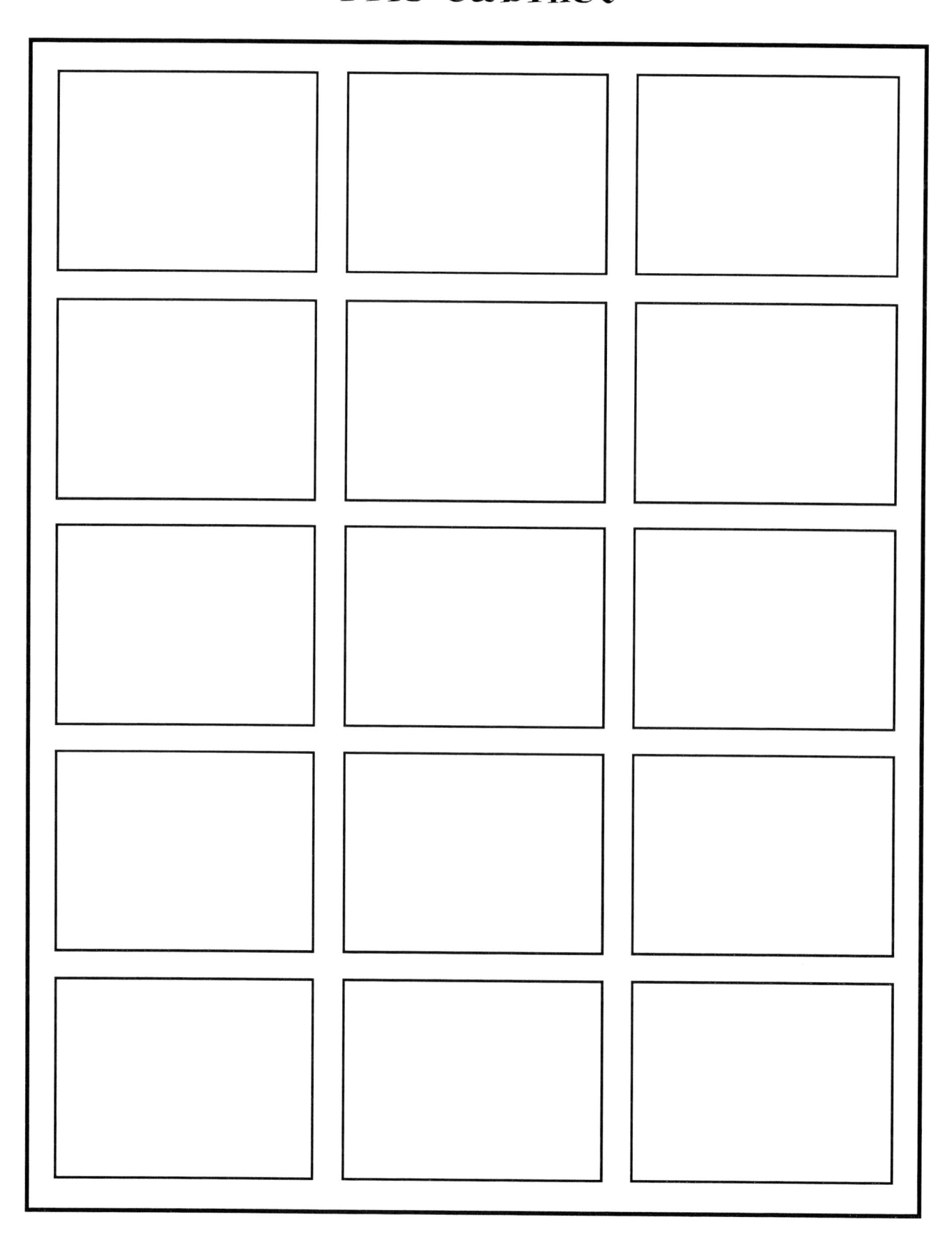

Three-Dimensional Space:

Floor Grid Games and More

Instructions for Making a Floor Grid

1. Cut a piece of masking tape approximately 4 ft. long and place it on the floor oriented vertically as shown below.

2. Using the first vertical tape line as a guide, cut and place four more 4 ft. pieces of tape approximately 1 ft. apart as shown.

3. Cut and place a 4 ft. piece of tape oriented horizontally as shown.

4. Using the first horizontal tape line as a guide, cut and place four more 4 ft. pieces of tape approximately 1 ft. apart as shown.

   When completed, you will have a floor grid with sixteen 1 ft. x 1 ft. squares. You may adjust the size of your floor grid to accommodate your treatment space and your client's needs.

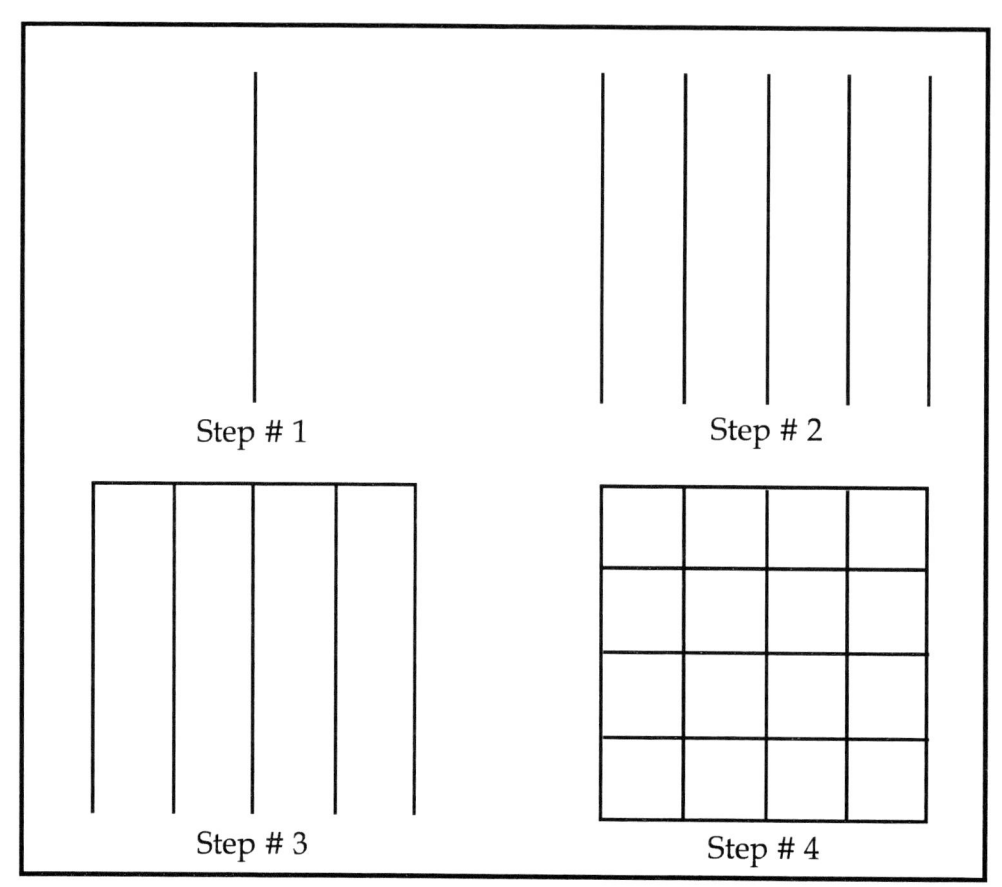

Table 3: Making a Floor Grid

Using Floor Grids

- When playing Floor Grid games, it is important to teach the child to face in the same direction throughout the game. This helps the child project directional concepts from her body to the environment more easily. A visual cue such as a wall clock or a poster can help the child stay oriented in the same direction.

- The lower left square of the floor grid always serves as the "starting square."

- Movement in the floor grid will be right, left, forward or backward.

- When moving to the right or left, teach the child to *sidestep*. This will ensure that she stays oriented correctly.

- Help the child count squares while moving. For example, say, "Go two squares forward, sidestep one square right."

Remote Control Robots

Purpose

To differentiate directional concepts in three-dimensional space. To follow directional instructions in three-dimensional space.

Materials

Masking tape

Procedure

- Using the tape, make a floor grid as described on page 104.

- Ask the child to pretend to be a robot. Tell the child, "Make-believe that you are my robot. You can only move when I tell you to. Start the game by standing in the starting square, and I will turn your power on."

- Once the child is standing in the starting square, say, "Now you must follow my instructions. I will tell you to move from square to square. I might tell you to go forward, backward, right or left. Make sure that you stay faced in the same direction."

- Continue by giving the robot directional instructions as in the example below:

    "Robot, hop two squares forward."

    "Robot, sidestep one square to the right."

    "Robot, jump one square forward."

    "Robot, tiptoe three squares backward."

    "Robot, heel-walk two squares forward."

    "Robot, frog-hop one square backward."

    "Robot, monster-stomp one square to the left."

- Direct the robot back to the starting square and "turn the power off" to end the game.

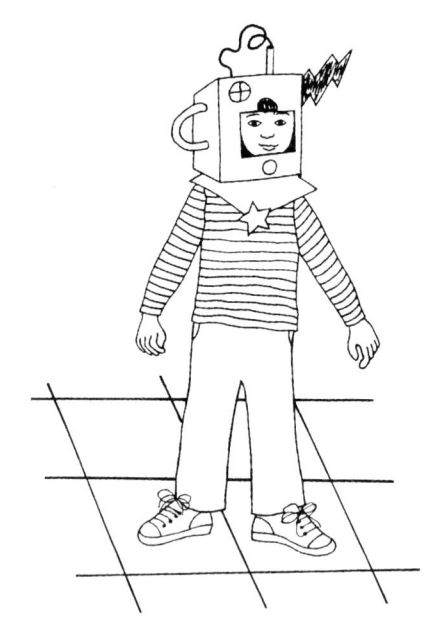

LEVEL 3—ENVIRONMENT AS A REFERENCE POINT

Observe

Does the child understand directional concepts relative to the floor grid? Can the child follow your directional instructions? Does the child turn around in the squares and become disoriented? If so, find a visual cue in the room to help the child orient his body relative to the grid. Say, for example, "Do you see the clock on the wall? When you are in the grid, make sure that you are always facing the clock." Notice if the child's responses are slow and tentative or quick and confident.

More Ideas

Make this activity more challenging by choosing two children to be robots. Position the robots so that they stand in their own starting squares facing one another. Use two diagonal corner squares of the floor grid for the starting points. Proceed by giving the robots the same directional instructions simultaneously.

Floor Grid Memory Match

Purpose

To differentiate directional concepts in three-dimensional space. To follow directional instructions in three-dimensional space. To practice visual memory and matching skills.

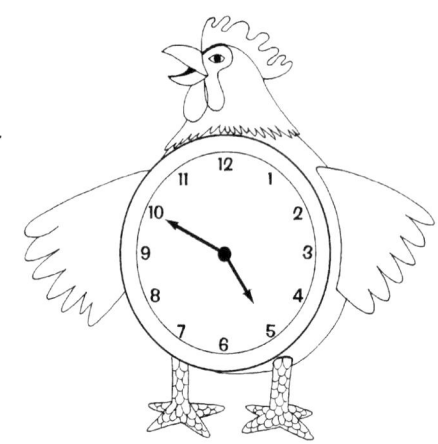

Materials

Masking tape and reproducible *Memory Match* pairs found on pages 110-117

Procedure

- Using the tape, make a floor grid as described on page 104.

- Photocopy the 8 *Memory Match* pairs. Cut along the dotted lines to separate the pairs into 16 separate pictures. If you wish, attach each picture to tagboard and laminate for durability. Mix up the 16 *Memory Match* pictures.

- Show the child the *Memory Match* pictures saying, "Look at these pictures. There are eight different pictures. Each picture has a match. Let's put them together in matching pairs."

- After you and the child have matched the pictures, discuss them. Say, "Let's talk about the pictures. What do you see in this picture? What is happening in this picture? Try to remember the pictures. Close your eyes and imagine the picture in your mind. Now we are ready to start the game."

- You and the child turn the 16 *Memory Match* pictures face down and mix them up. Place one picture face down in each floor grid square.

- Continue instructing the child by saying, "Walk to the floor grid and stand in a square. You can stand in any square. Make sure that you stay faced in the same direction."

- When the child gets to the square say, "Now pick up the picture and turn

LEVEL 3—ENVIRONMENT AS A REFERENCE POINT

it over. Which picture do you see? What is happening in the picture?"

- After the child describes the picture aloud, tell him or her to return it to the floor grid square face up so that the picture is visible. Tell the child to "Remember where the picture is."

- Continue the game by saying, "Now go stand in another square. Pick up a new picture and turn it over. Which picture do you see? What is happening in the picture? Does it match the first picture?"

- If the pictures match, allow the child to remove them from the floor grid. If they do not match, instruct the child to turn them face down again. Play continues until the child locates all eight matching pairs of *Memory Match* pictures.

Observe

This game is a "moving" version of the classic board game, *Memory*. The floor grid helps the child orient the position of the pictures in space. The floor grid also allows the child to orient her body while moving through space. Does the child have difficulty orienting in space? Can the child recall the location of the pictures? Help her by giving directional instructions such as, "Try the picture in the upper right corner square" or "Sidestep one square to the left. See if that picture matches." Remind the child to face the same way throughout the game. If necessary, use a visual cue such as a wall clock as a reminder.

More Ideas

Use the *Memory Match* picture cards to work on language skills. Play an adapted version of the board game, *Memory*. Arrange the picture pairs face down on a table in the grid configuration. As the game is played, have the child describe each picture as she turns it face up. Work on sentence formation, pronouns, verbs, etc. Explain the similarities and differences between playing the game at a table and on the floor grid.

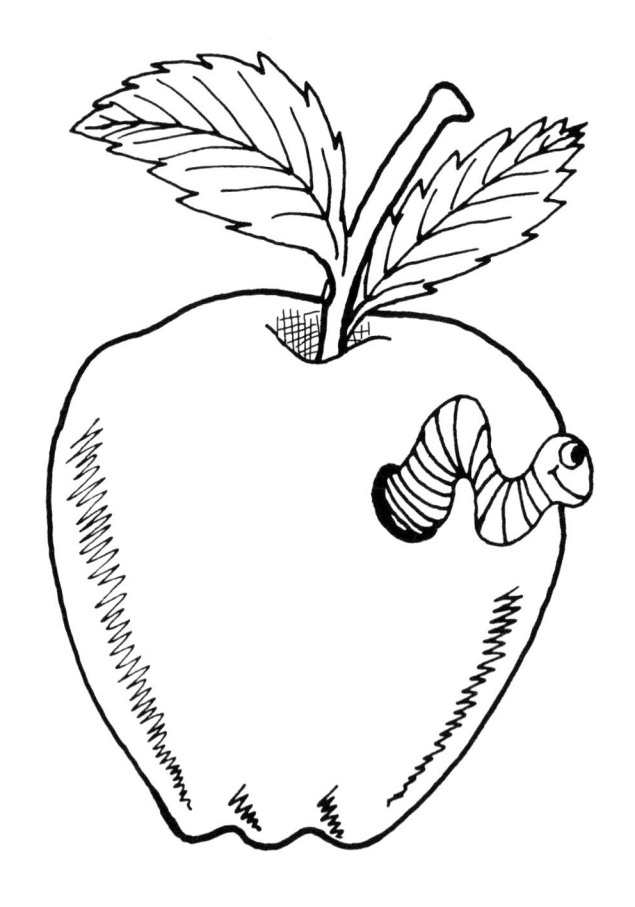

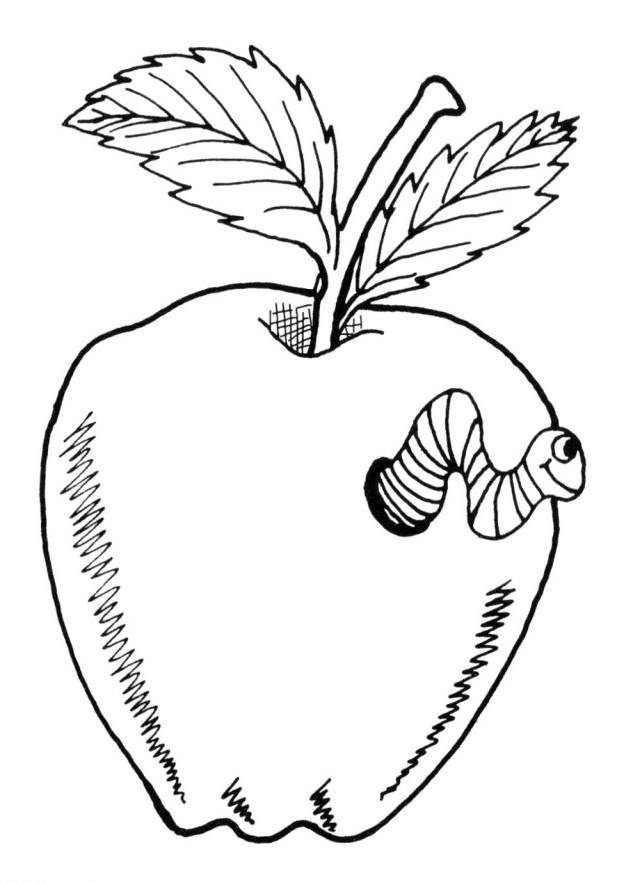

Reproducible. Copyright © 1999 Imaginart International, Inc.

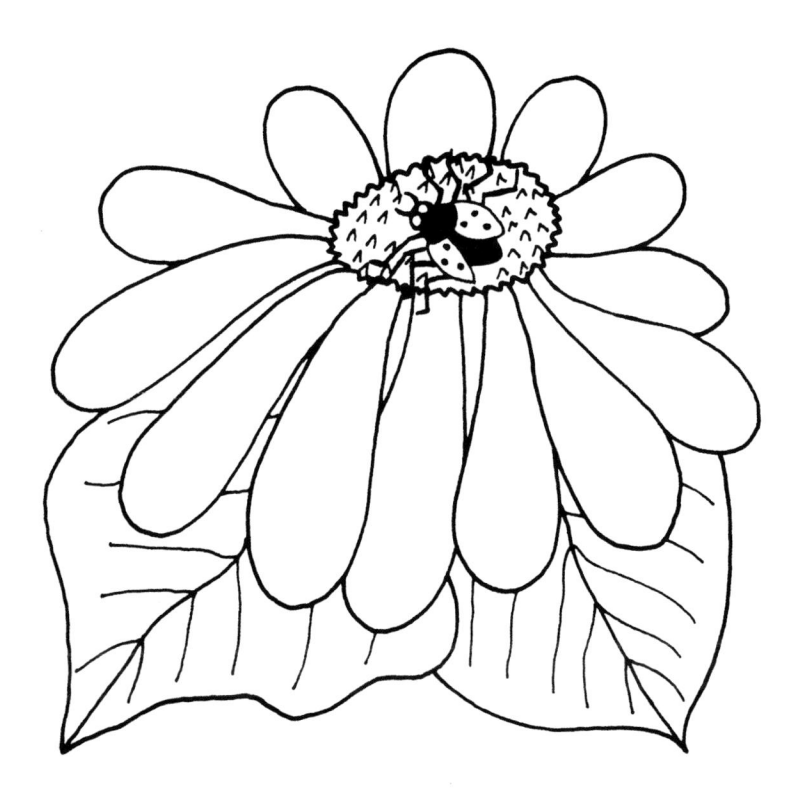

Reproducible. Copyright © 1999 Imaginart International, Inc.

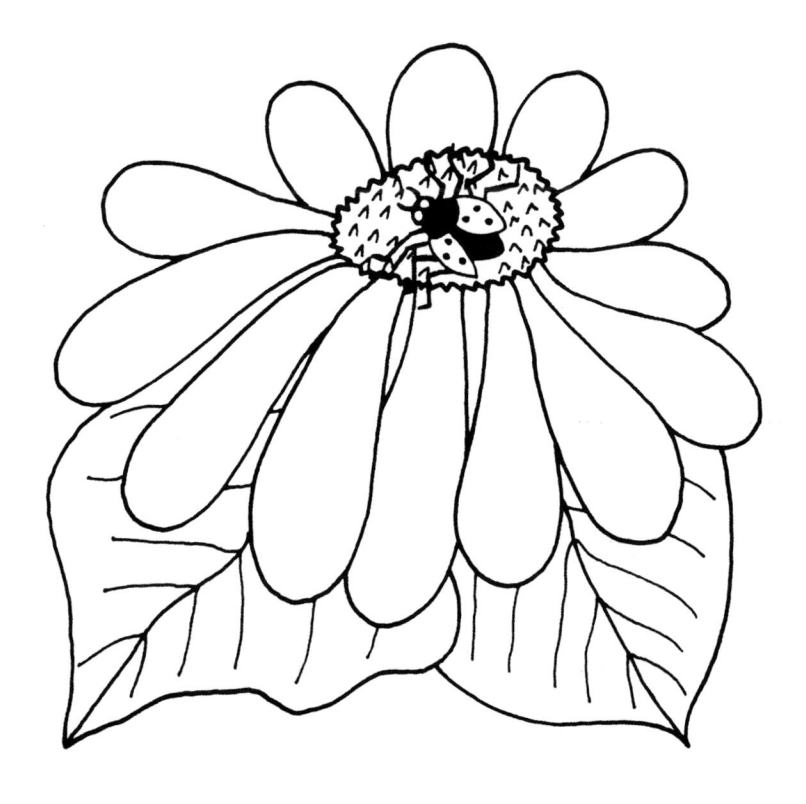

111

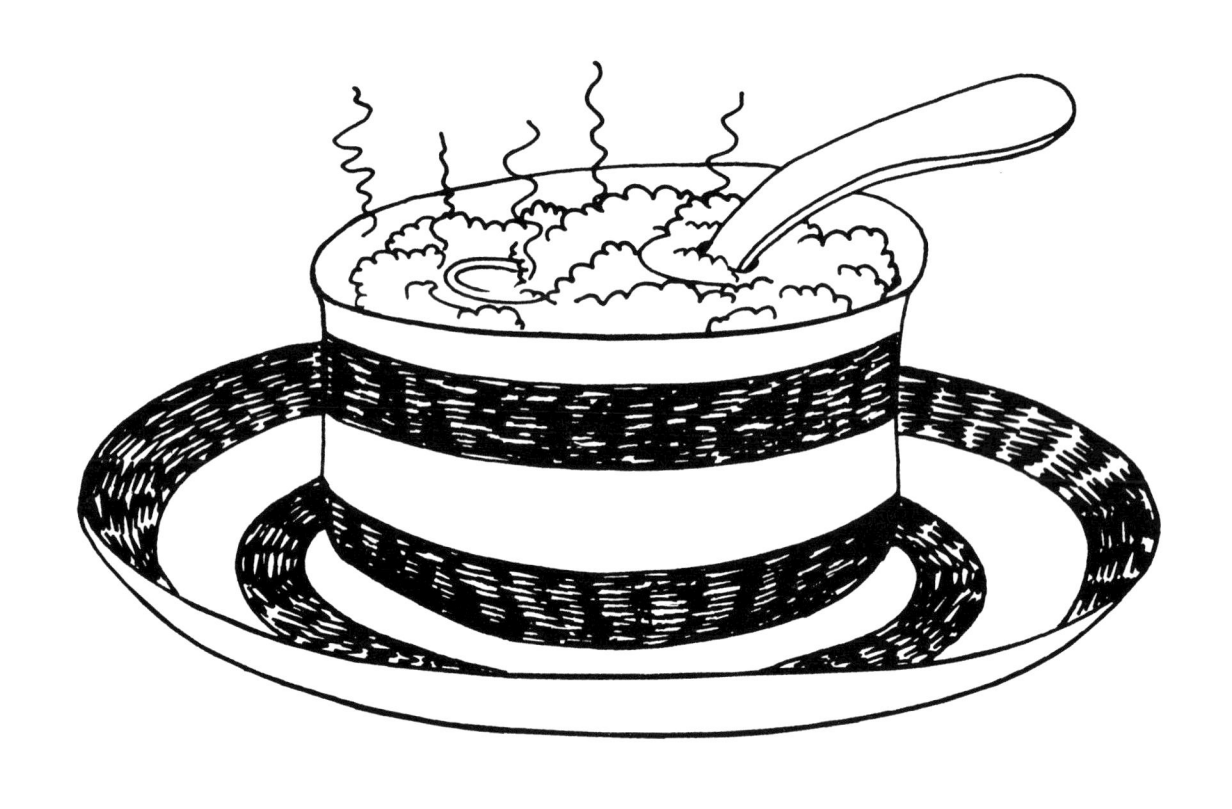

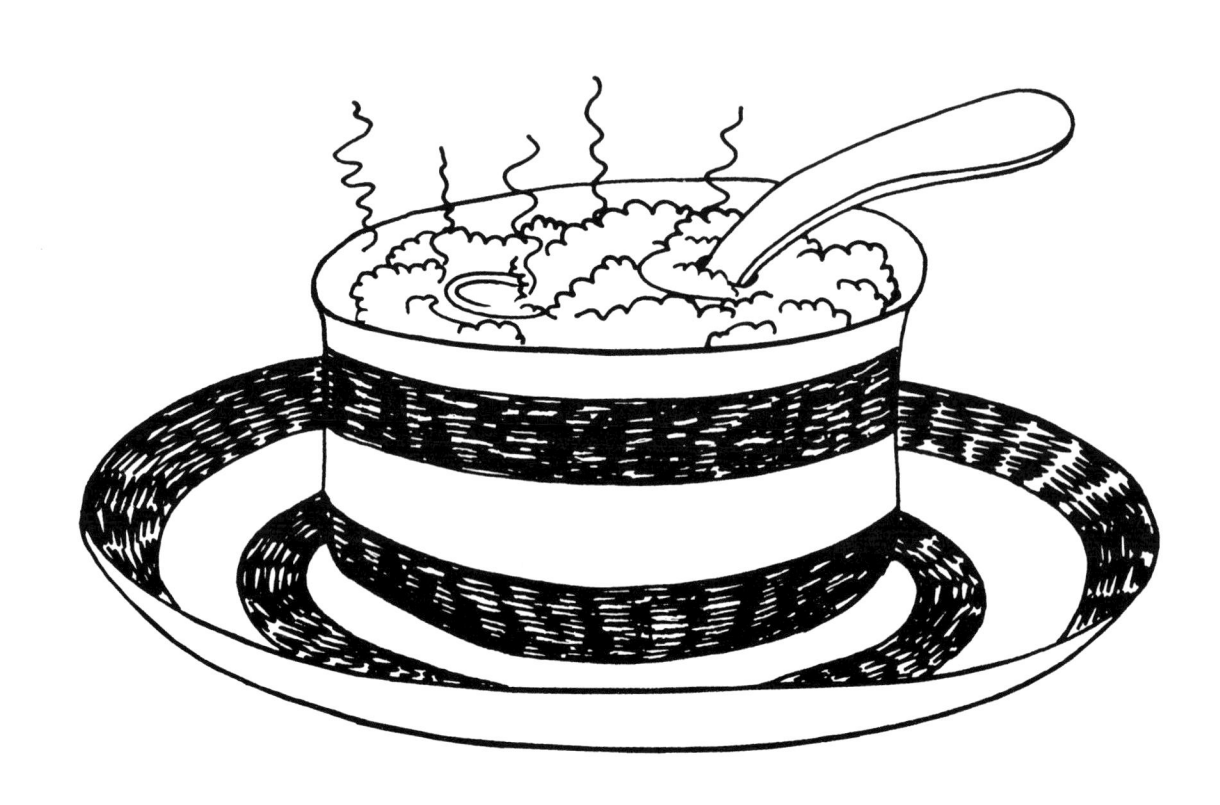

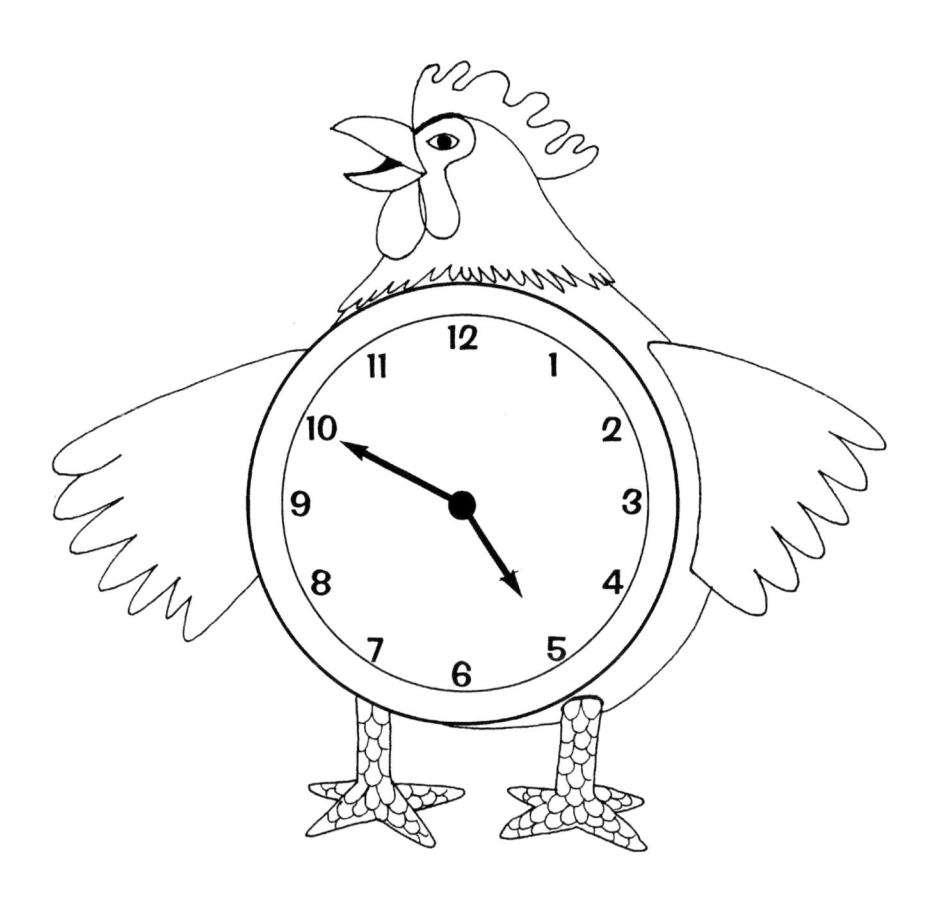

Reproducible. Copyright © 1999 Imaginart International, Inc.

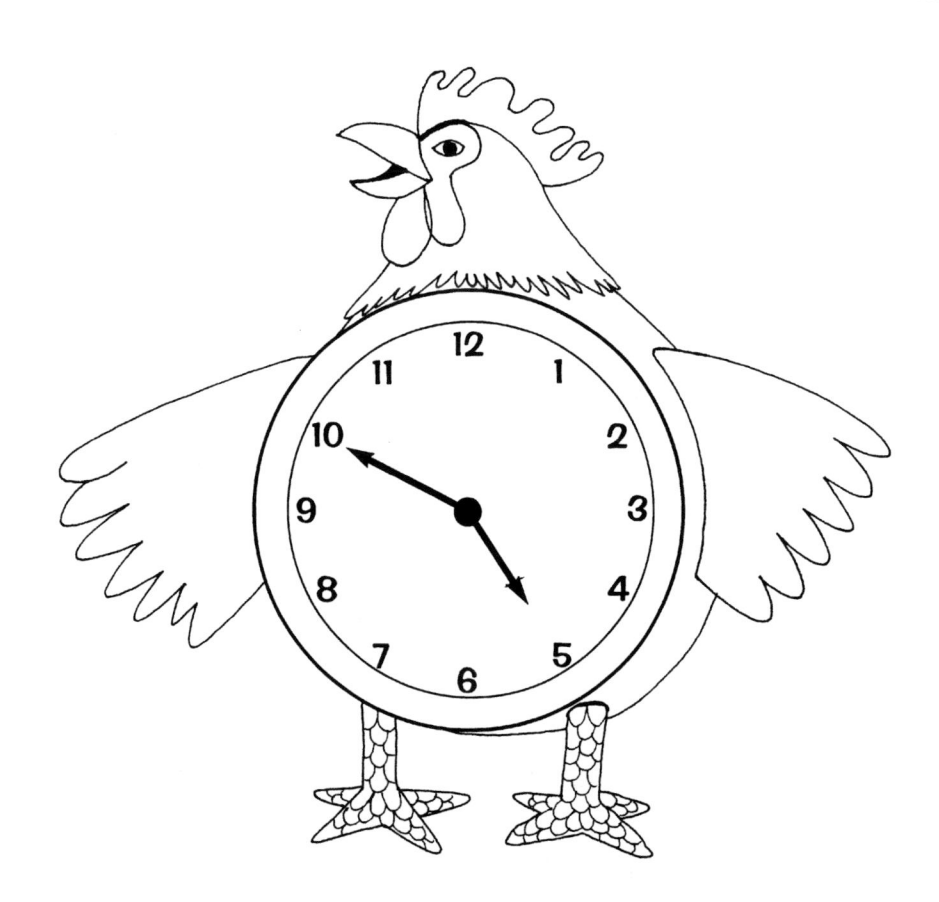

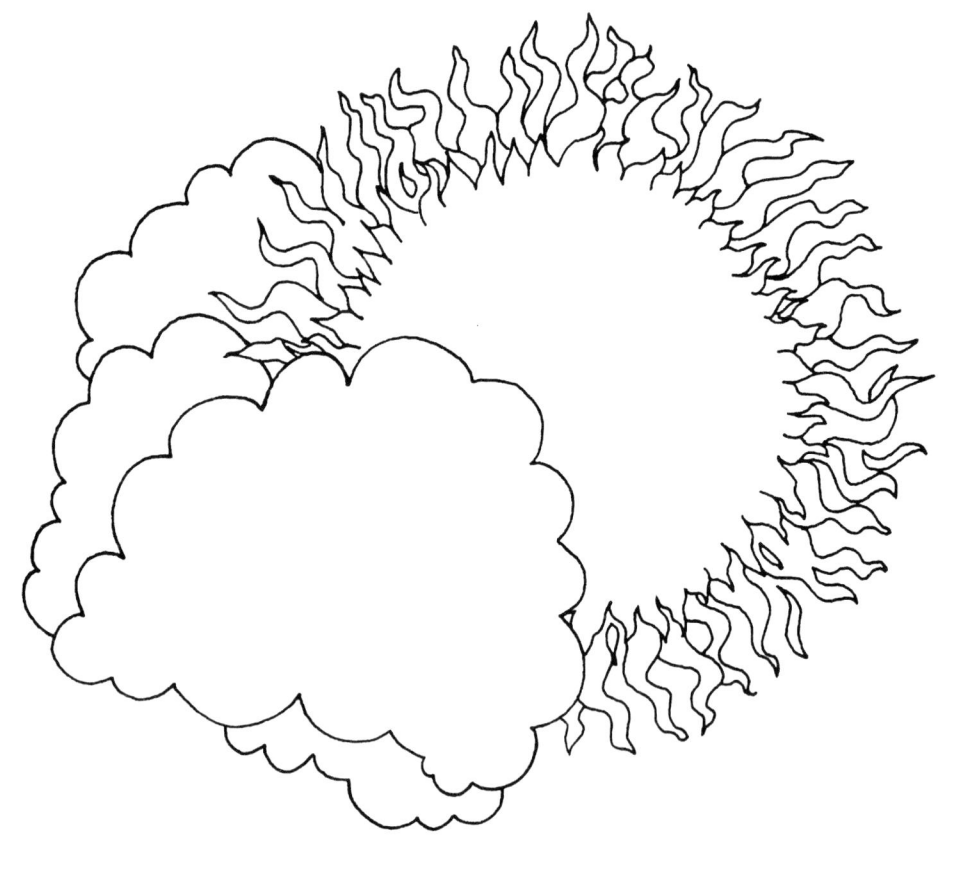

Reproducible. Copyright © 1999 Imaginart International, Inc.

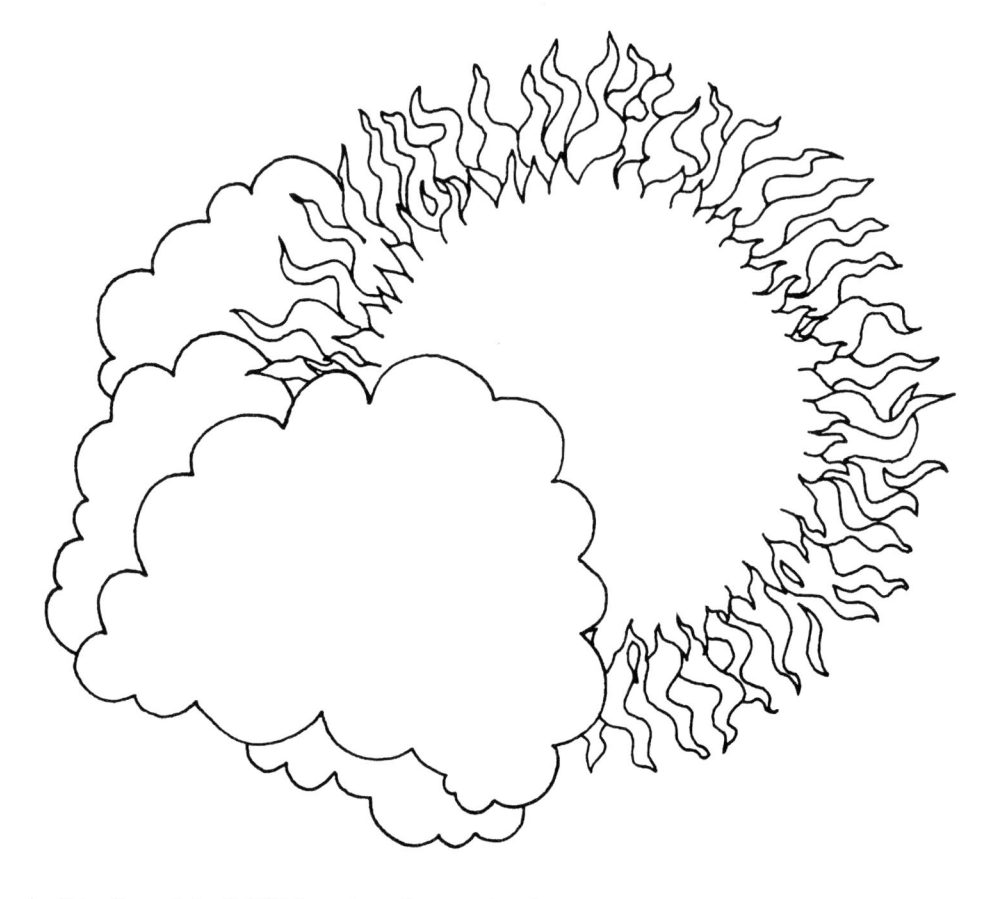

114

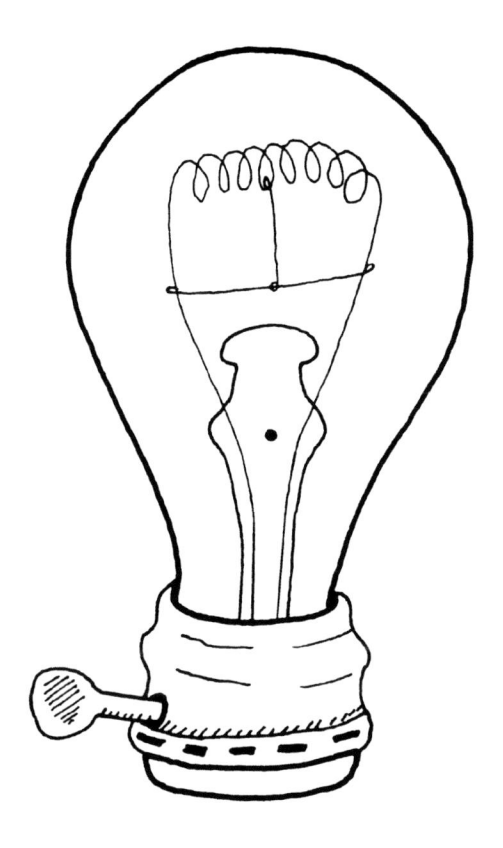

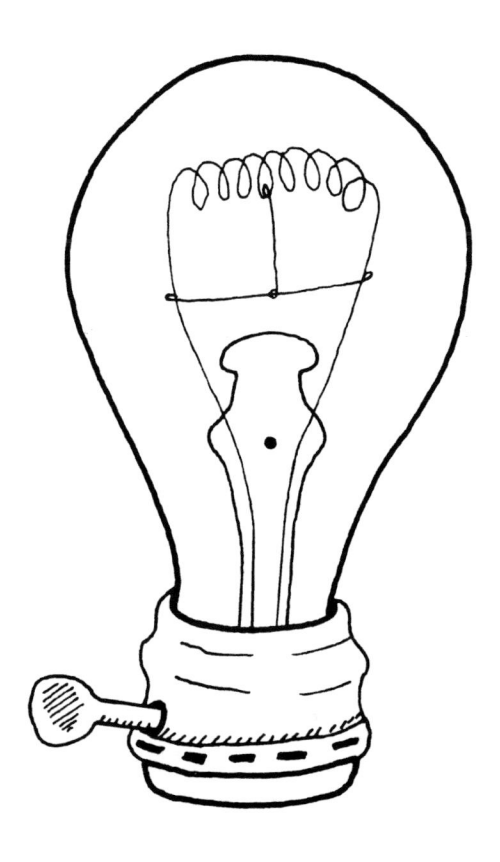

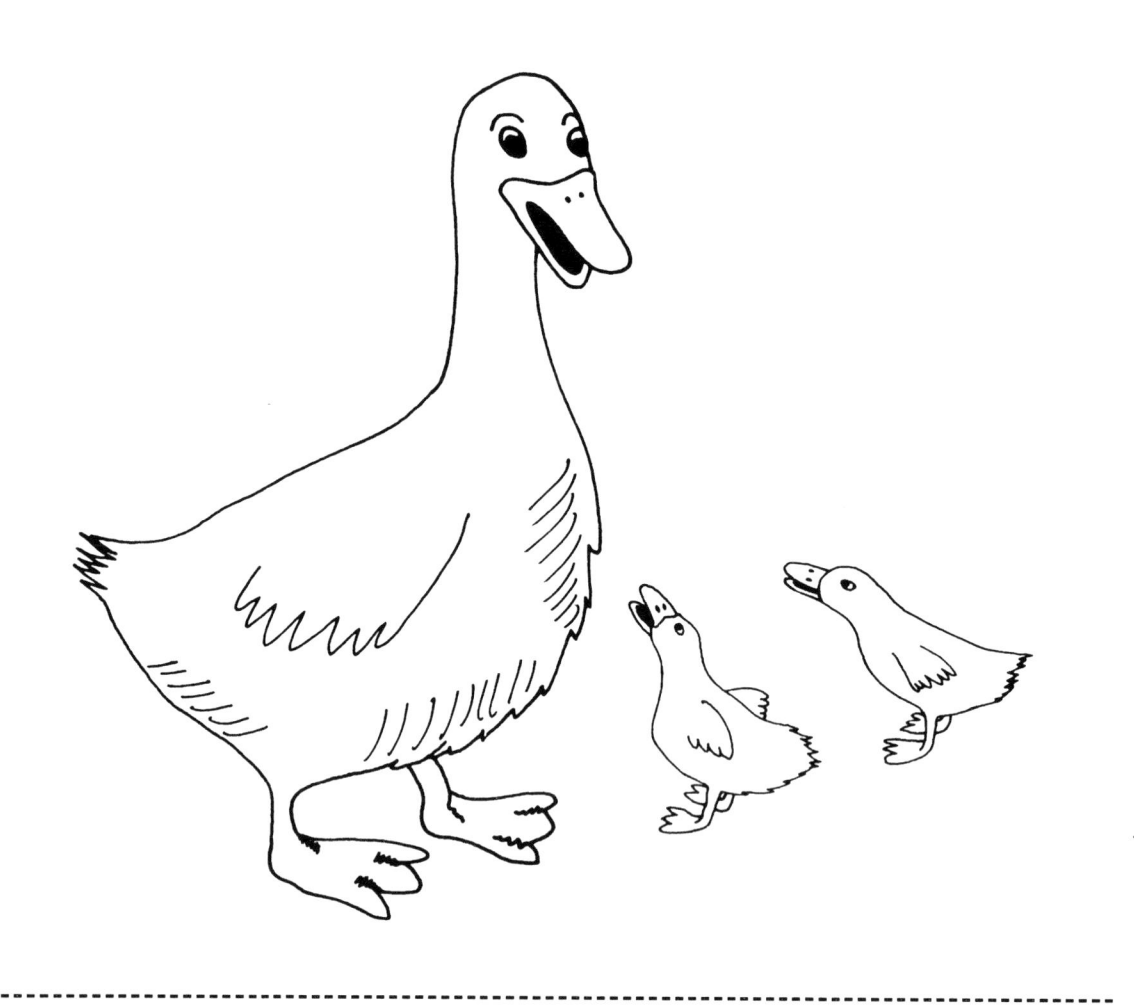

Reproducible. Copyright © 1999 Imaginart International, Inc.

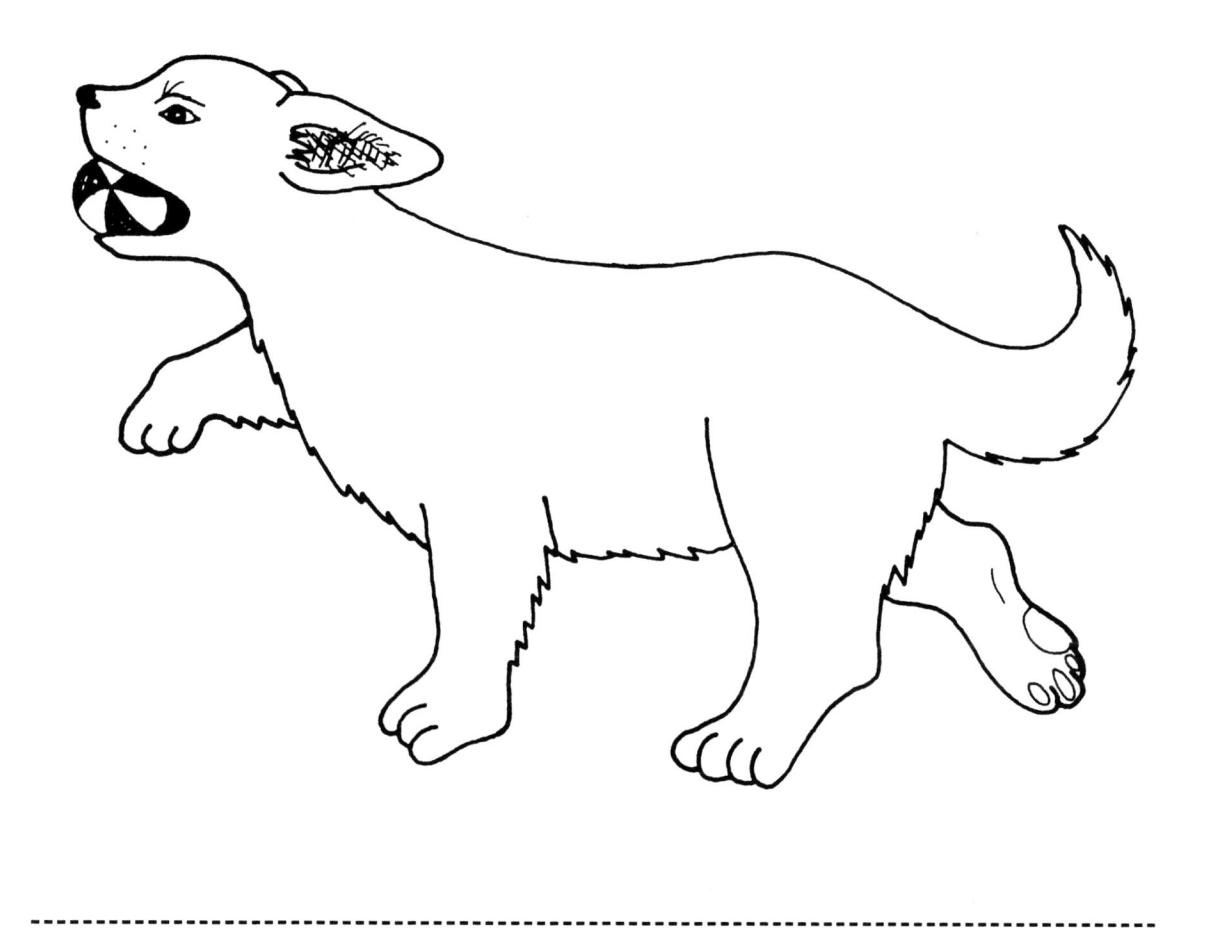

117

Sticker Hunt
Floor Grid Game

Purpose

To differentiate directional concepts in two-dimensional space and three-dimensional space. To project directional concepts from a two-dimensional surface to a three-dimensional environment.

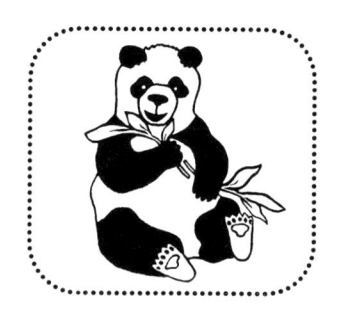

Materials

Masking tape, 16 index cards, stickers, 16-square grid map on page 206 and a marker

Procedure

- Using the tape, make a floor grid as described on page 104.

- Before starting the game, place an index card in each square. Turn over one of the index cards and put a sticker on it. Then replace it face down so the sticker cannot be seen. Remember the location of this "secret sticker card."

- Use the 16-square grid map to mark the location of the secret sticker card. Draw an "X" in the square with the sticker card. Make a map from the starting square to the "X" by drawing vertical and horizontal lines from square to square. Now you are ready to begin the game.

- Tell the child, "You are going on a sticker hunt. There is a sticker hidden under one of these cards in the floor grid. Your job is to find the secret sticker card."

- Give the child the map and explain, "Use this map to find the secret sticker card. The map has grid lines and squares just like the floor grid."

- Instruct the child to stand in the starting square, holding the map so that it is oriented correctly. Tell the child, "Now use the map to guide you from square to square. When you get to the square with the "X," pick up the card and see if you have found the secret sticker. Remember to stay faced in the same direction as you move."

LEVEL 3—ENVIRONMENT AS A REFERENCE POINT

Observe

Can the child project the directional concepts from the map to three-dimensional space? Can the child orient her body relative to both the map and the grid? If the child has difficulty orienting in space, use extra visual cues and give additional instructions as follows: "Do you see the clock on the wall? When you are in the grid, make sure that you are always facing the clock. When you need to move to the right or left, side-step so that you are always facing the same way. Hold the map so that it matches the grid at all times."

More Ideas

Ask the child to read the map aloud while moving from square to square by saying "right, left, forward or backward."

Allow the child to hide the secret sticker and draw the map for you to follow.

LEVEL 3—ENVIRONMENT AS A REFERENCE POINT

Animal Parade
Floor Grid Game

Purpose

To differentiate directional concepts in two-dimensional and three-dimensional space. To project directional concepts from a two-dimensional surface to a three-dimensional environment.

Materials

Masking tape, reproducible *Animal Parade* pictures found on page 122-125, black marker and a completed *Animal Parade* grid map as described on page 82

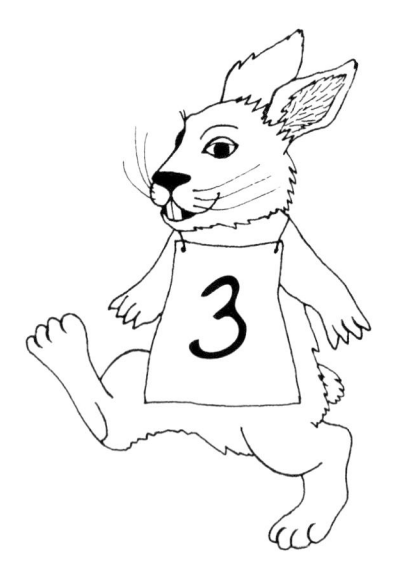

Procedure

- Using tape, make a floor grid as described on page 104.

- Before the game begins, photocopy the 8 *Animal Parade* pictures. Cut along the dotted lines to separate the pictures. Using the black marker, number each animal from 1 to 8. If you wish, attach each picture to tagboard and laminate for durability.

- Referring to the child's completed *Animal Parade* grid map, place the numbered animal pictures in the corresponding floor grid squares. Now you are ready to start the game.

- Tell the child, "These animals are going to march in a parade. Each animal has a number. Your job is to go to each animal in correct number order so they can march in the parade."

- Give the child the completed grid map and explain, "Here is the map that you made before. The map has grid lines and squares just like the floor grid."

- Instruct the child to stand in the starting square, holding the map so that it is oriented correctly. Tell the child, "Now use the map to go to each animal in order from 1 to 8. Remember to stay faced in the same direction as you move."

LEVEL 3—ENVIRONMENT AS A REFERENCE POINT

Observe

Does the child understand numerical sequencing? Can the child project the directional concepts from the map to the three-dimensional space? Can the child orient her body relative to both the map and the floor grid? If the child has difficulty orienting in space, use extra visual cues and give additional instructions as follows: "Do you see the clock on the wall? When you are in the grid, make sure that you are always facing the clock. When you need to move right or left, sidestep so that you are always facing the same way. Hold the map so that it matches the grid at all times. Count the squares as you move."

More Ideas

Ask the child to read the map aloud while moving from square to square by saying, "right, left, forward or backward."

Allow the child to color the animal pictures.

To play the game again, simply use a blank *Animal Parade* grid to draw a new map.

Make the activity more challenging by asking the child to find the animals in order without a map. The child must tell you which way she is moving—right, left, forward or backward.

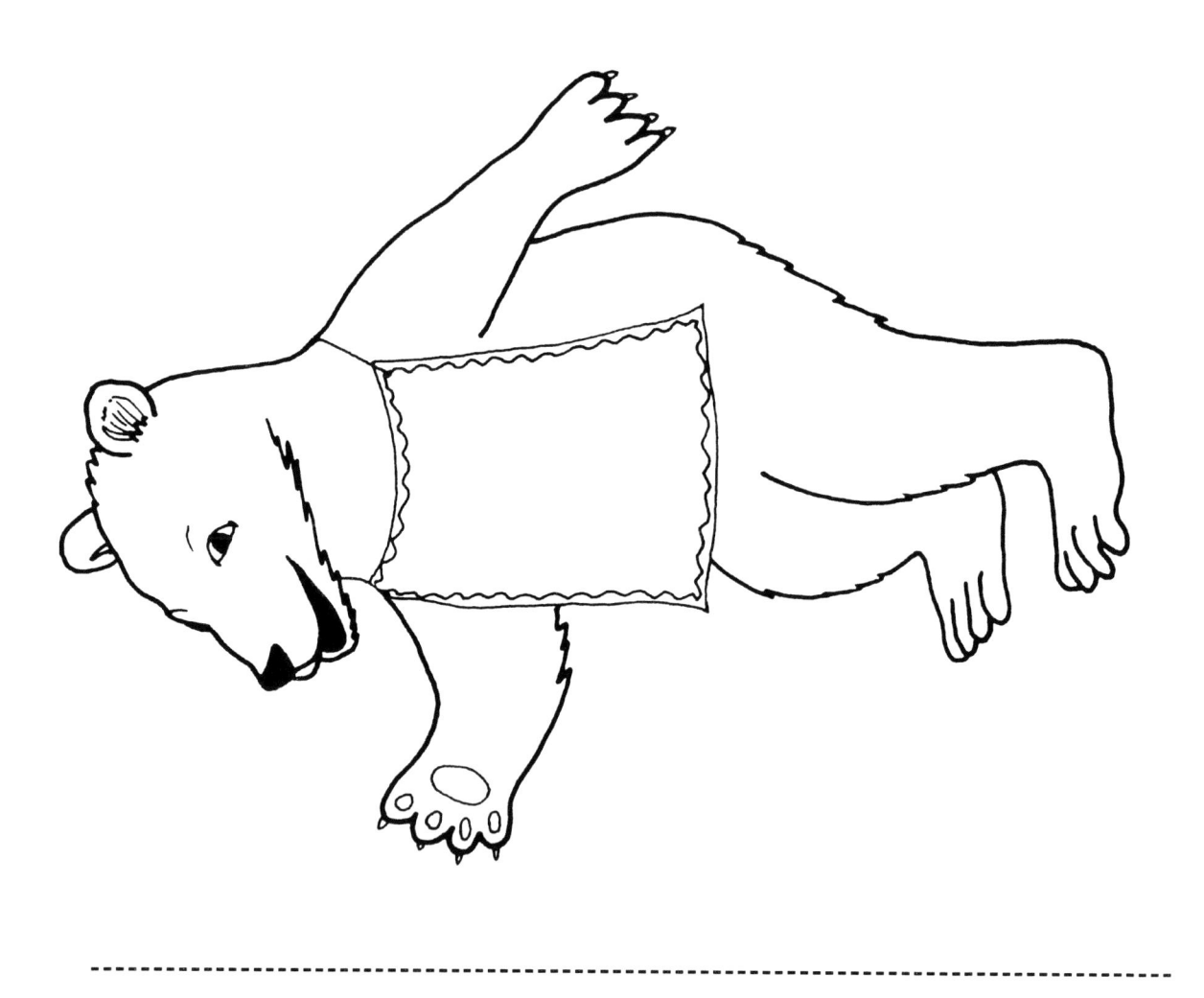

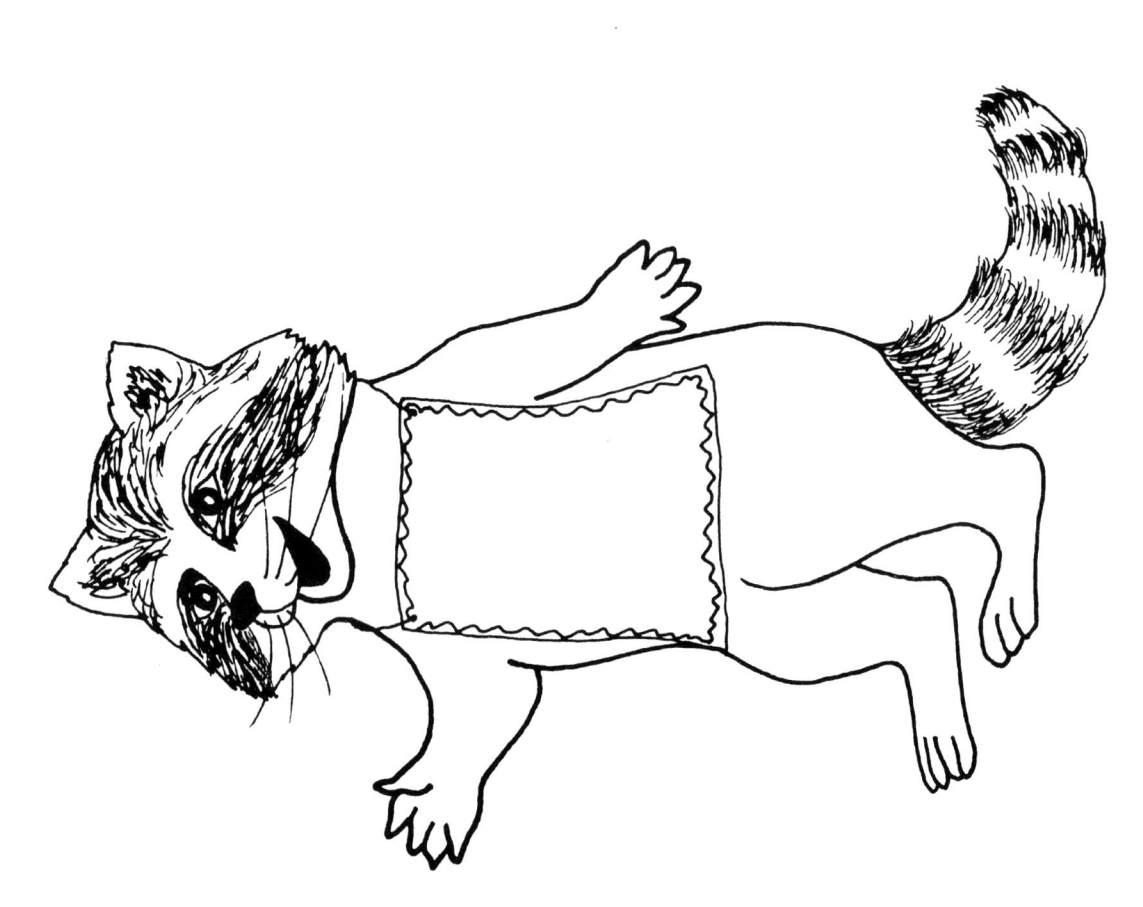

Reproducible. Copyright © 1999 Imaginart International, Inc.

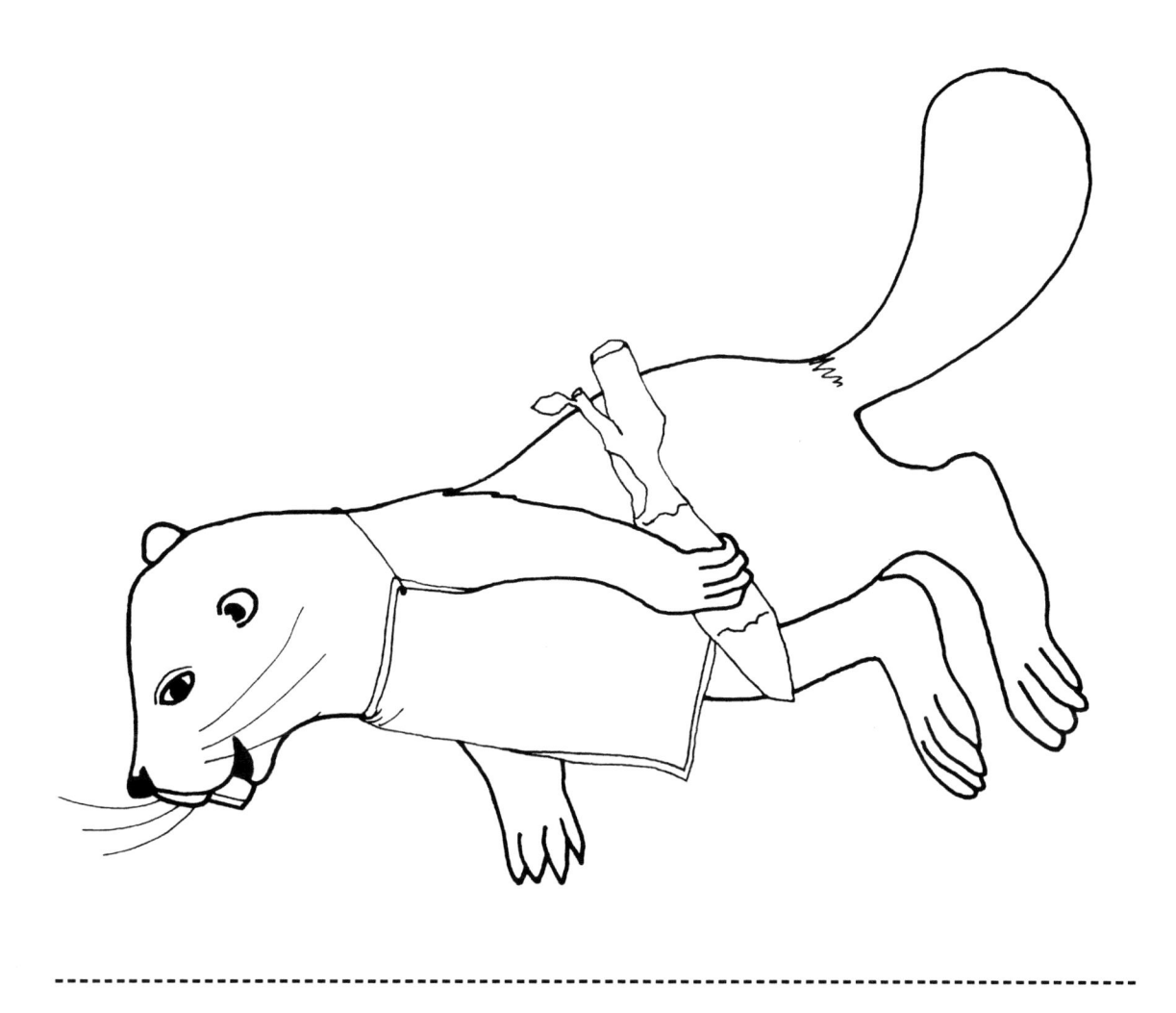

Reproducible. Copyright © 1999 Imaginart International, Inc.

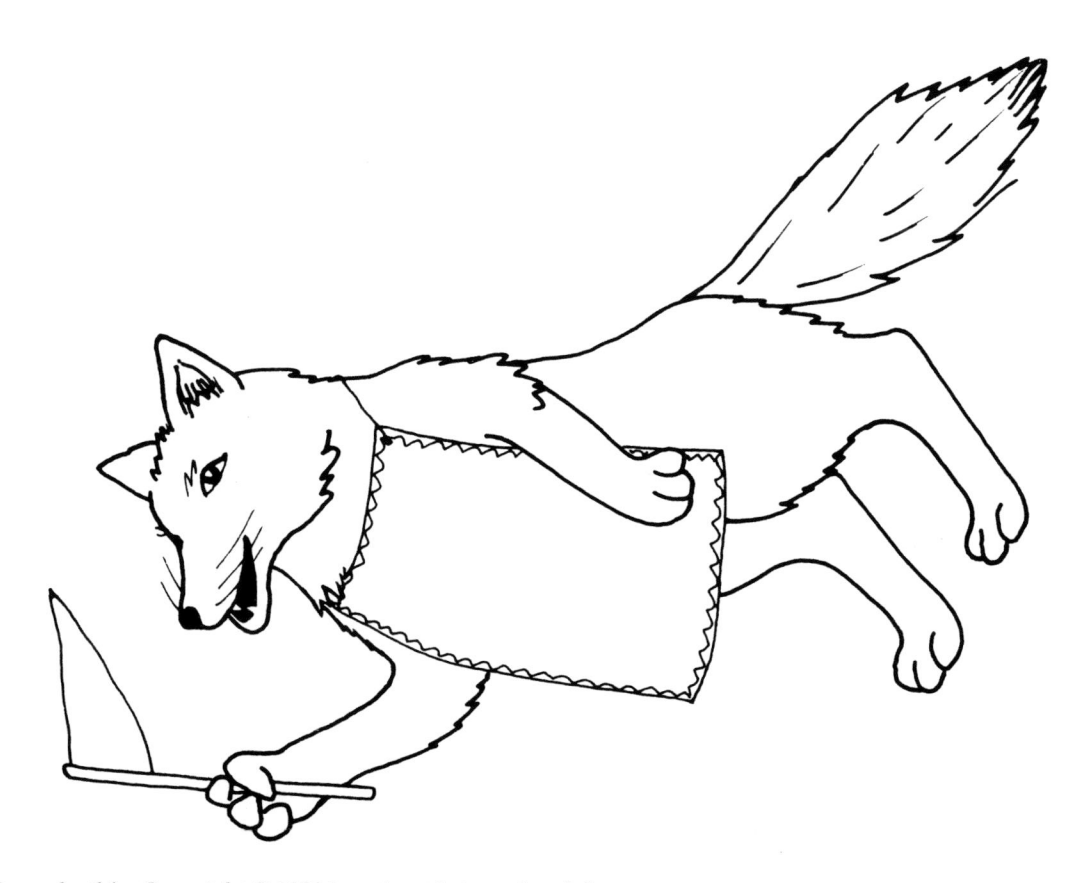

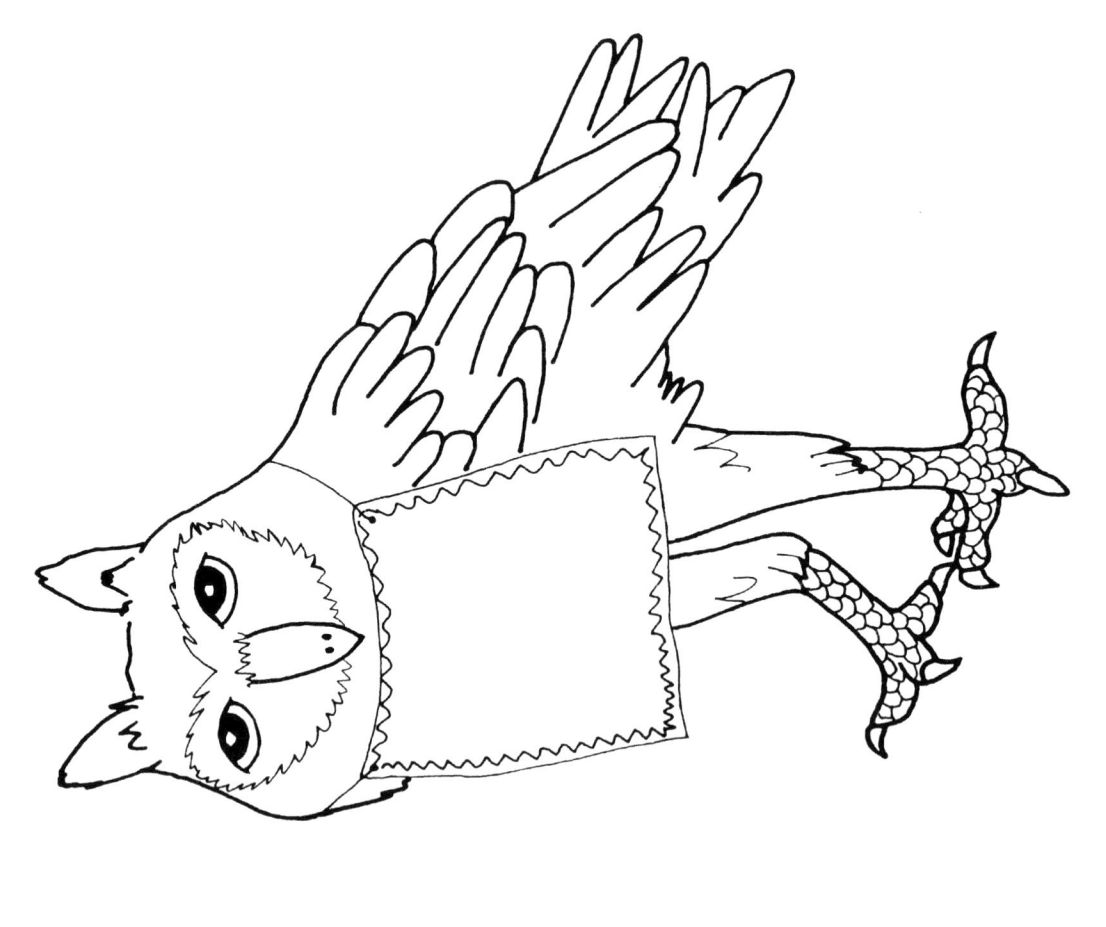

Reproducible. Copyright © 1999 Imaginart International, Inc.

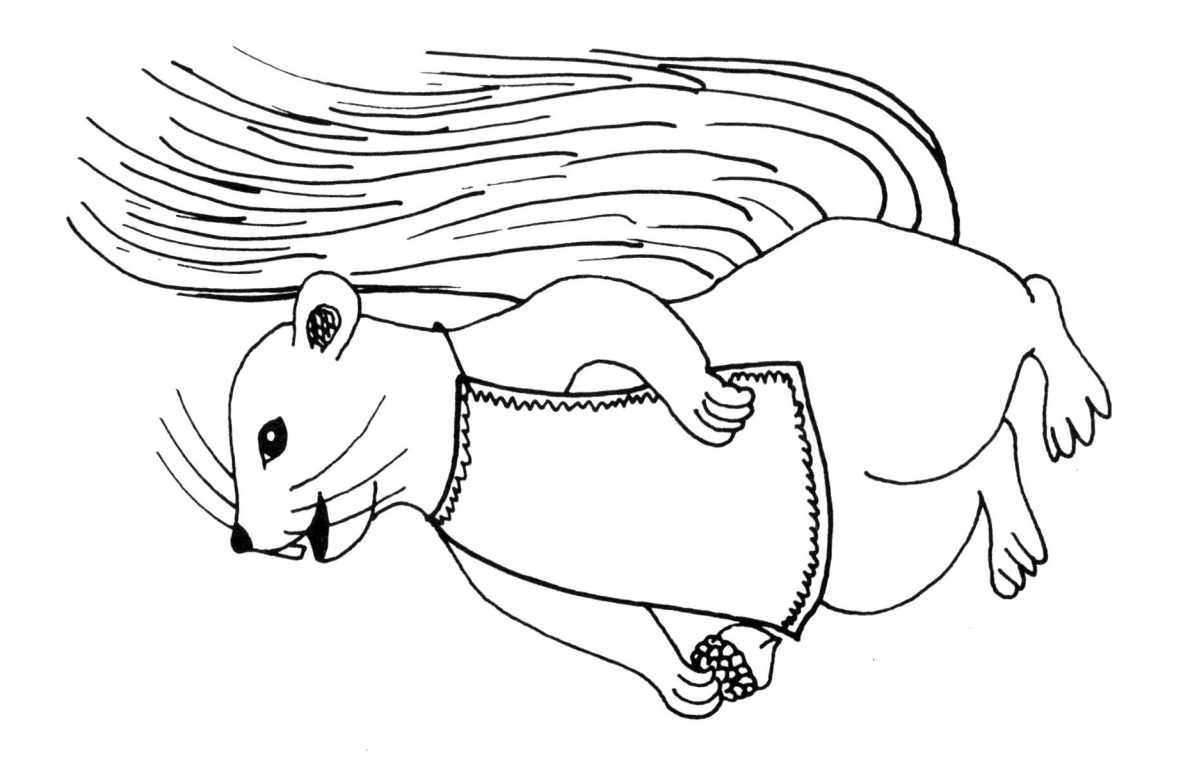

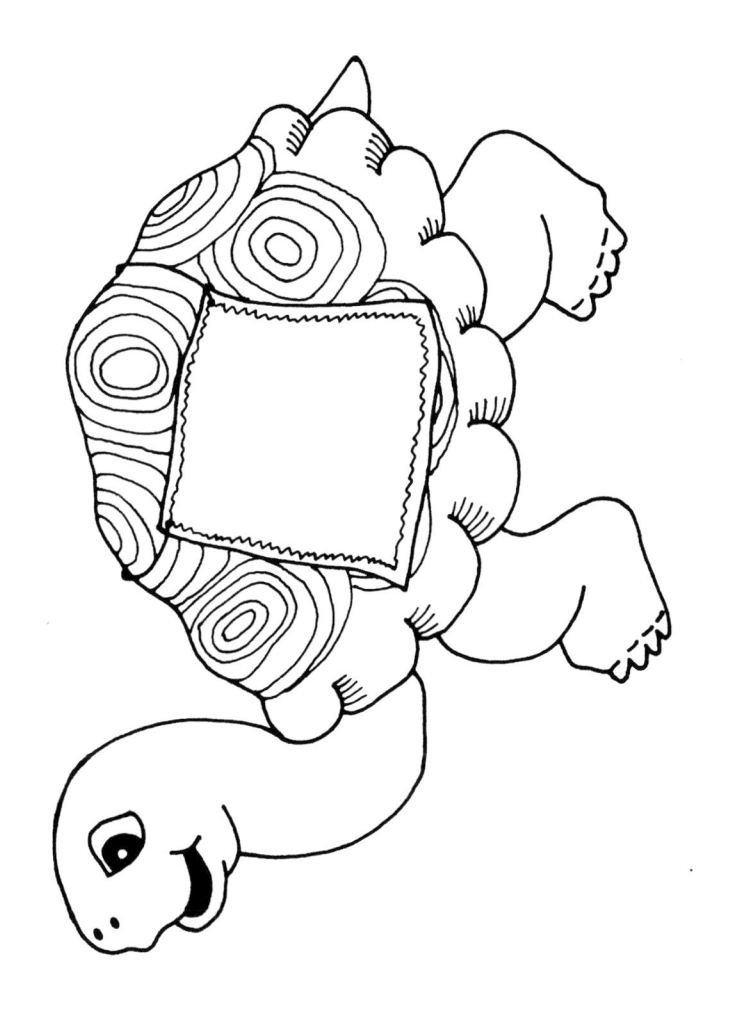

Reproducible. Copyright © 1999 Imaginart International, Inc.

Mixed-Up Socks
Floor Grid Game

Purpose

To differentiate directional concepts in two-dimensional and three-dimensional space. To project directional concepts from a two-dimensional surface to a three-dimensional environment.

Materials

Masking tape, reproducible *Mixed-Up Socks* pictures found on page 128-131, black marker and a completed *Mixed-Up Socks* grid map as described on page 85

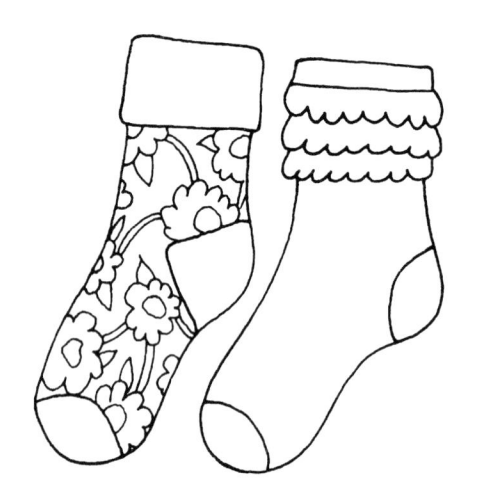

Procedure

- Using tape, make a floor grid as described on page 104.

- Before the game begins, photocopy the 8 *Mixed-Up Socks* pictures. Cut along the dotted lines to separate the pictures. If you wish, attach each picture to tagboard and laminate for durability.

- Referring to the child's completed *Mixed-Up Socks* grid map, place the socks in the corresponding floor grid squares. Now you are ready to start the game.

- Tell the child, "These socks are all mixed up. Your job is to find the socks that look the same and match them into pairs."

- Give the child the completed grid map and explain, "Here is the map that you made before. The map has grid lines and squares just like the floor grid."

- Instruct the child to stand in the starting square, holding the map so that it is oriented correctly. Tell the child, "Now use the map to go to the matching socks. Follow the lines on the map. Remember to stay faced in the same direction as you move."

LEVEL 3—ENVIRONMENT AS A REFERENCE POINT

Observe

Does the child understand the concept of matching? Can the child project the directional concepts from the map to the three-dimensional space? Can he orient his body relative to both the map and the floor grid? If the child has difficulty orienting in space, use extra visual cues and give additional instructions as follows: "Do you see the clock on the wall? When you need to move right or left, sidestep so that you are always facing the clock. Hold the map so that it matches the grid at all times. Count squares as you move."

More Ideas

Ask the child to read the map aloud while moving from square to square by saying, "right, left, forward or backward."

Allow the child to color the sock pictures.

To play the game again, simply use a blank *Mixed-Up Socks* grid, page 87, to draw a new map.

Use real pairs of socks to play the game. Mix up the socks and place them in the floor grid squares. Make the activity more challenging by asking the child to find the matching pairs without a map. The child must tell you which way he is moving—right, left, forward or backward while finding the pairs.

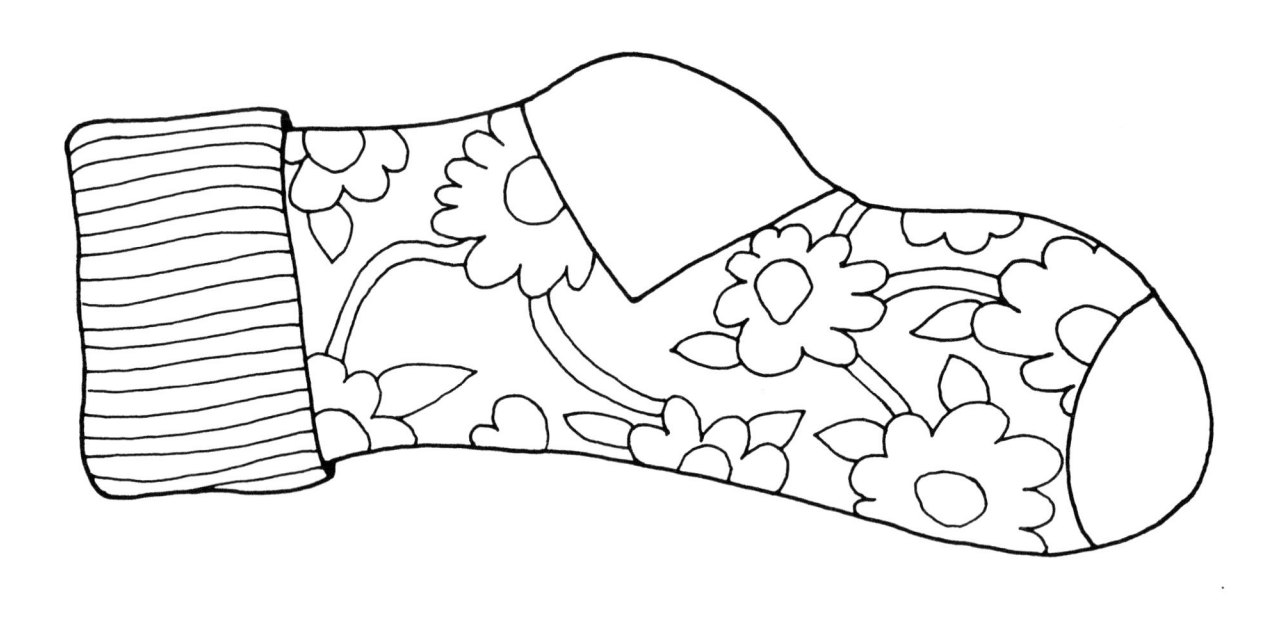

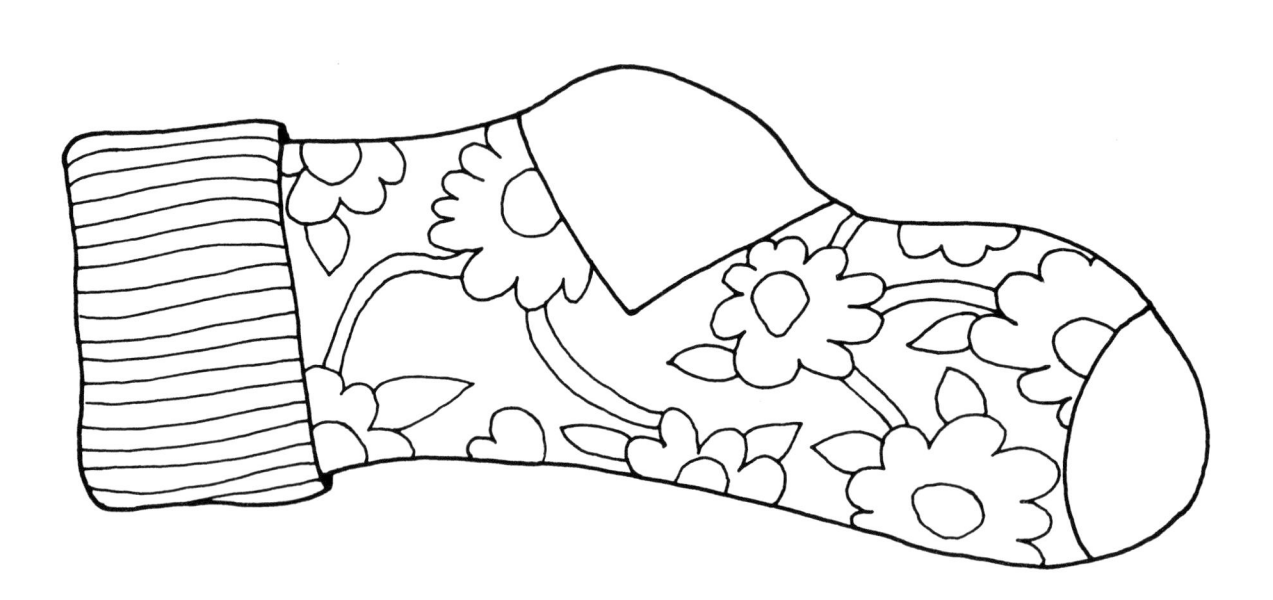

Reproducible. Copyright © 1999 Imaginart International, Inc.

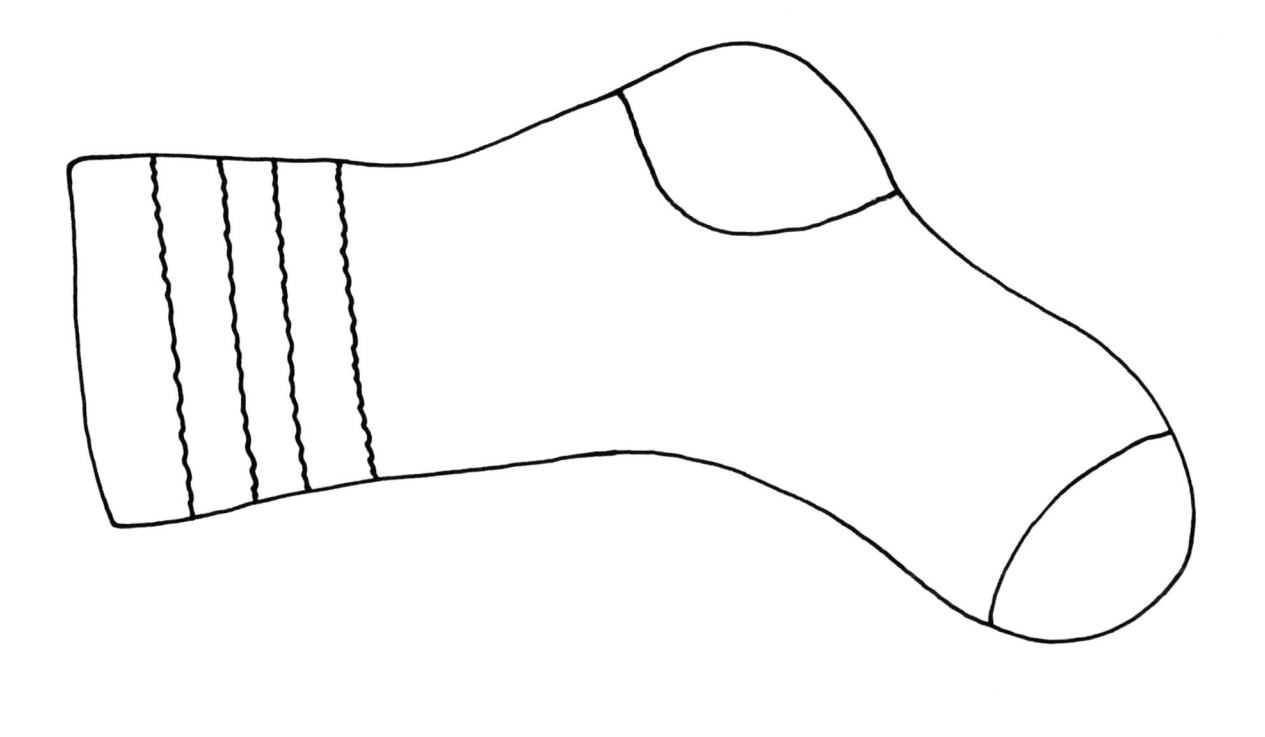

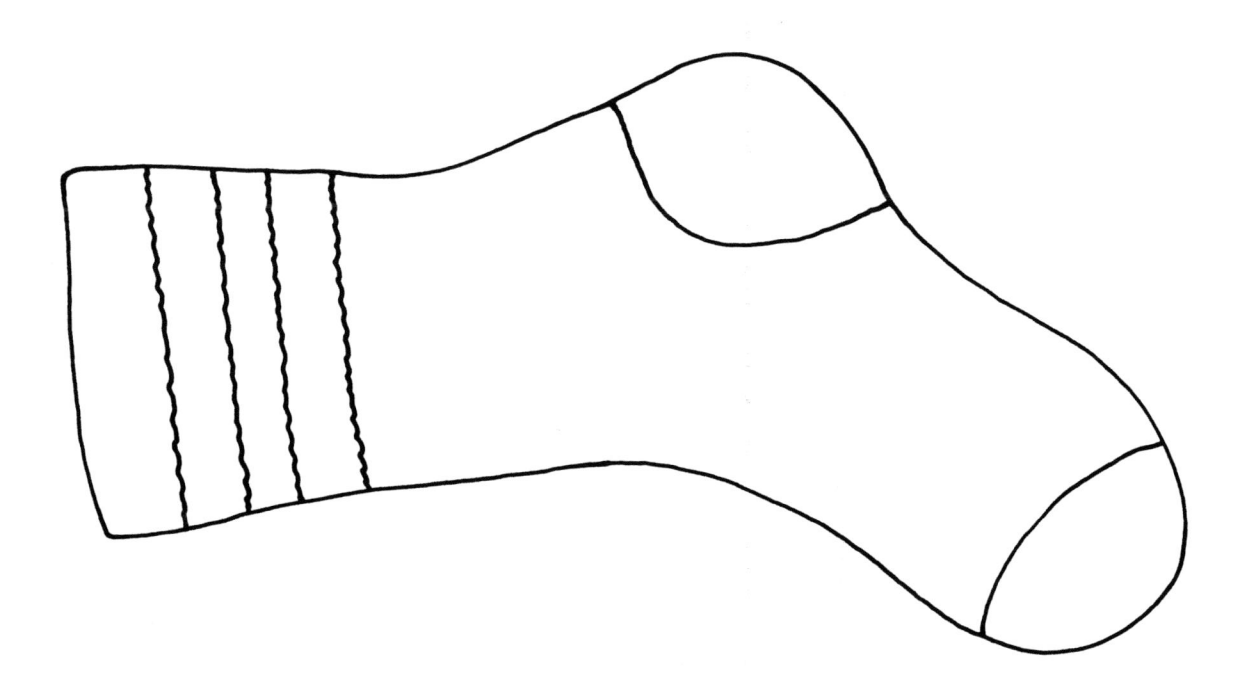

Reproducible. Copyright © 1999 Imaginart International, Inc.

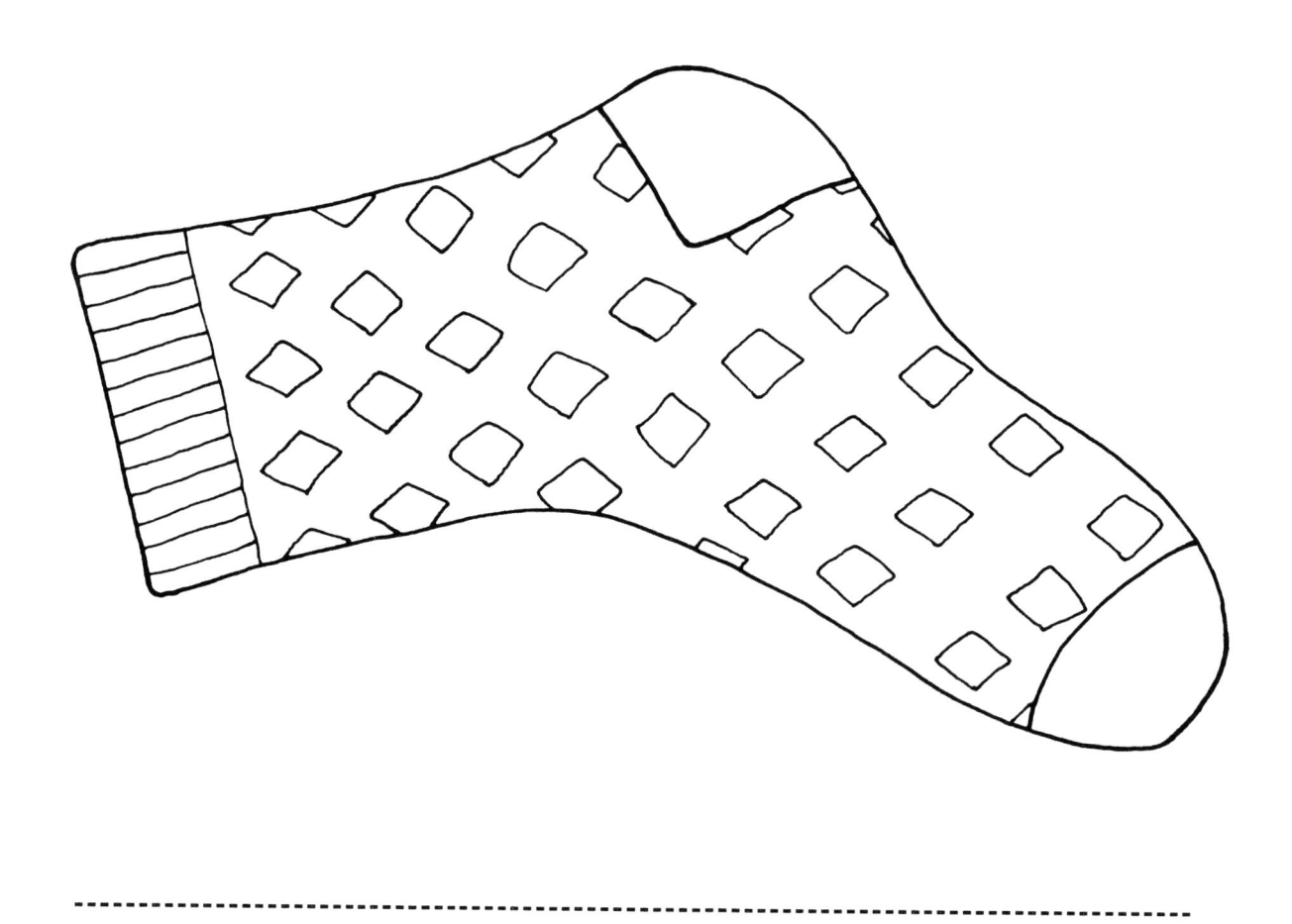

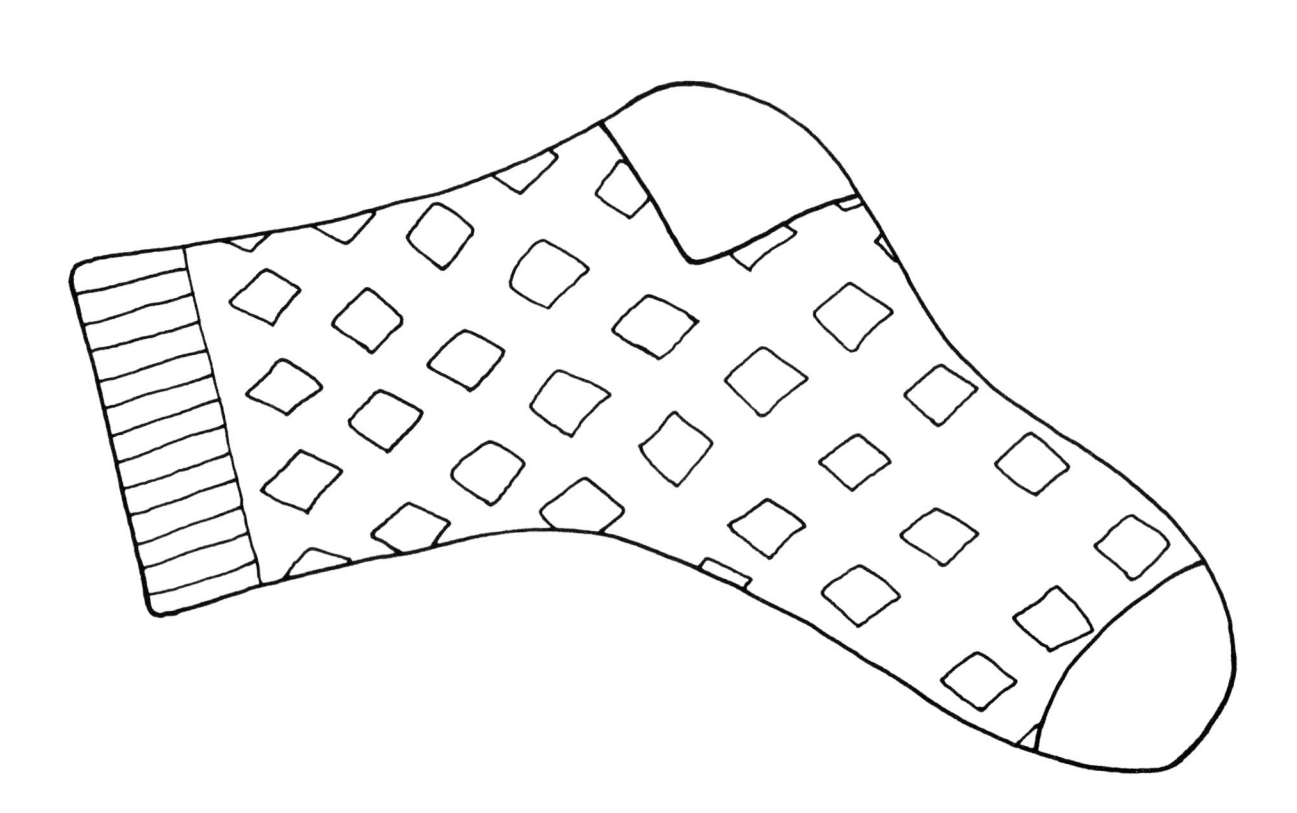

Reproducible. Copyright © 1999 Imaginart International, Inc.

130

131

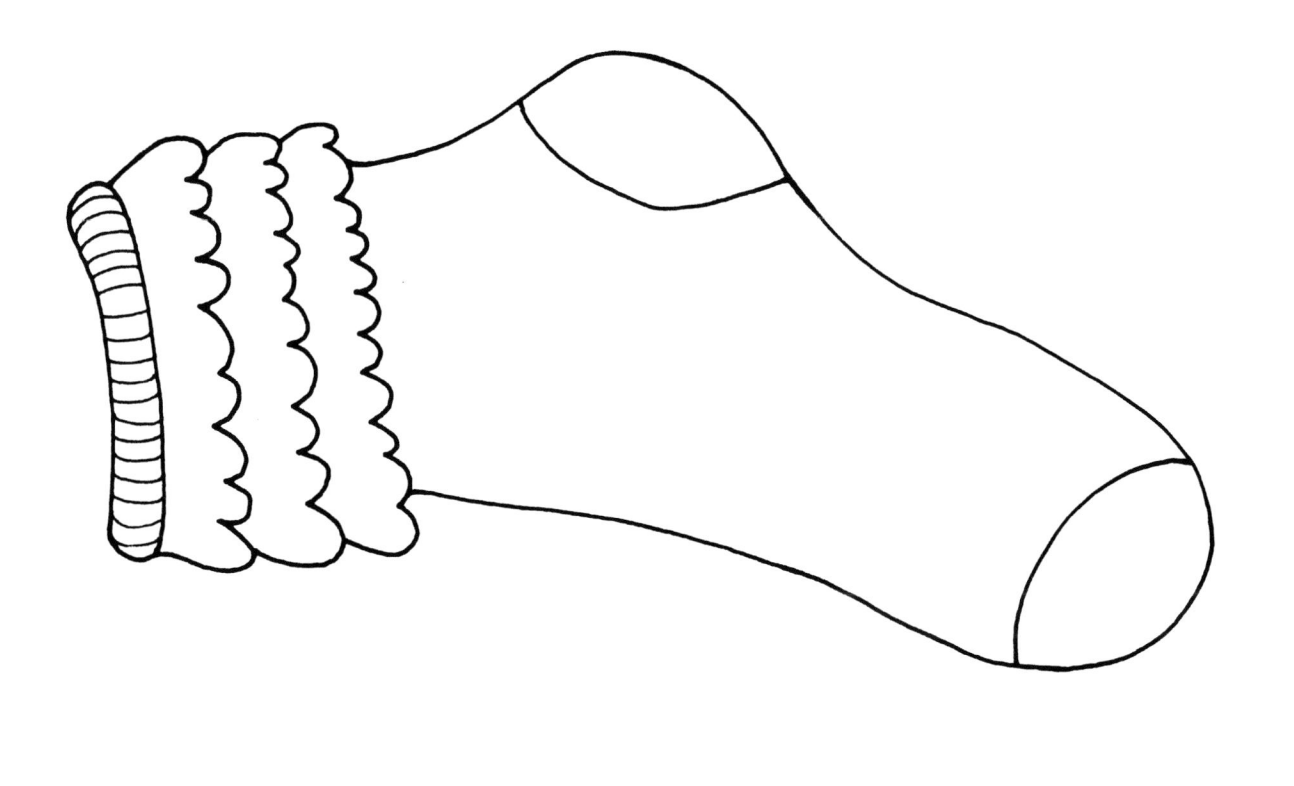

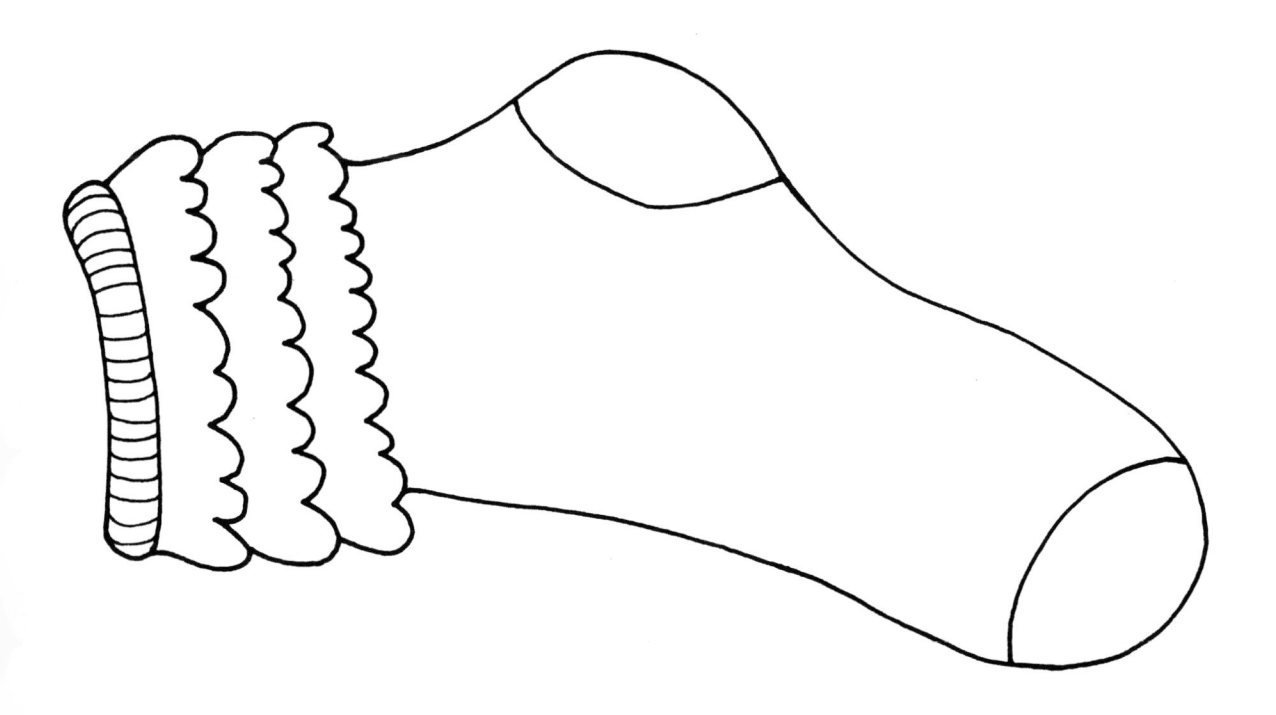

Mail Delivery
Floor Grid Game

Purpose

To differentiate directional concepts in two-dimensional and three-dimensional space. To project directional concepts from a two-dimensional surface to a three-dimensional environment.

Materials

Masking tape, reproducible *Mail Delivery* envelopes found on pages 134-137, a black marker and a completed *Mail Delivery* grid map as described on page 88

Procedure

- Using tape, make a floor grid as described on page 104.

- Before the game begins, photocopy the 8 *Mail Delivery* envelopes. Cut along the dotted lines to separate the pictures. Referring to the child's completed *Mail Delivery* grid map, print a name on each of the envelopes and place them in the corresponding floor grid squares. Now you are ready to begin the game.

- Tell the child, "These envelopes are for your friends (or classmates or family). Your job is to find each envelope in correct alphabetical order. After you have found them all, you can deliver them to your friends."

- Give the child the completed grid map and explain, "Here is the alphabetical list and map that you made before. The map has grid lines and squares just like the floor grid."

- Instruct the child to stand in the starting square, holding the map so that it is oriented correctly. Tell the child, "Now use the map to go to each envelope in alphabetical order. Remember to stay faced in the same direction as you move."

Observe

Does the child understand alphabetical order? Can the child project the directional concepts from the map to the three-dimensional space? Can the child orient her body relative to both the map and the floor grid? If she has difficulty orienting in space, use extra visual cues and give additional instructions as follows: "Do you see the clock on the wall? When you need to move right or left, sidestep so that you are always facing the clock. Hold the map so that it matches the grid at all times. Count squares as you move."

More Ideas

Ask the child to read the map aloud while moving from square to square by saying, "right, left, forward or backward."

Allow the child to decorate the envelopes.

To play the game again, simply use a blank *Mail Delivery* grid, page 90, to draw a new map.

Make the activity more challenging by asking the child to find the envelopes in order without a map. The child must tell you which way she is moving—right, left, forward or backward.

Use real envelopes to play the game.

Practice writing real addresses on the envelopes.

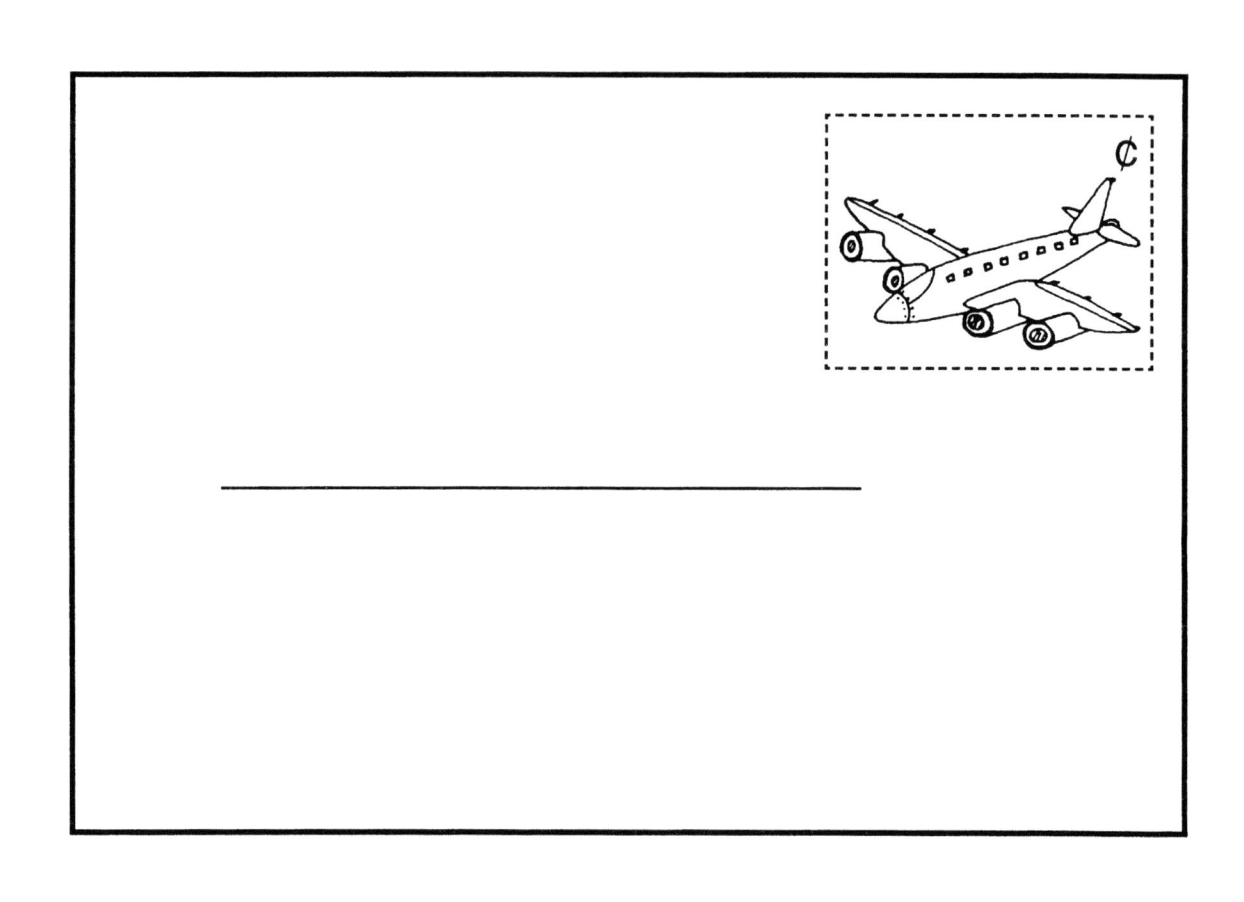

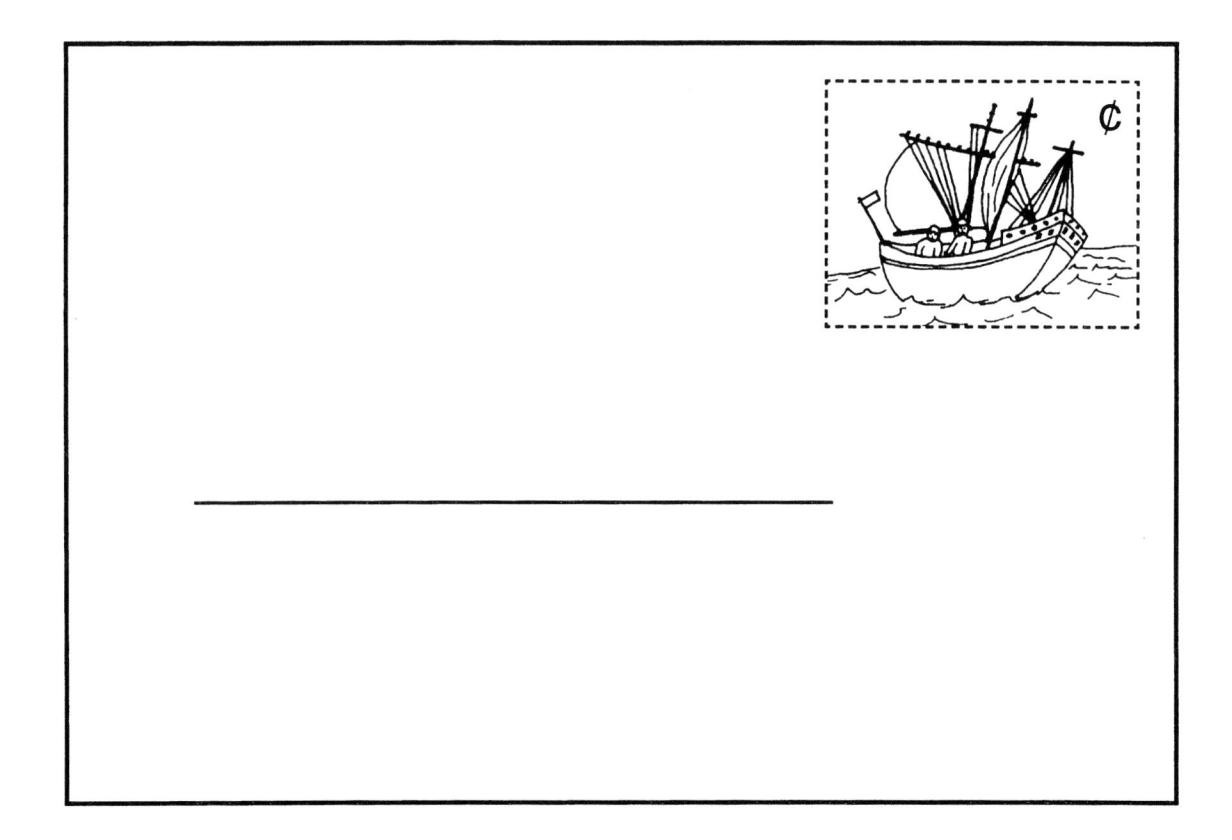

Reproducible. Copyright © 1999 Imaginart International, Inc.

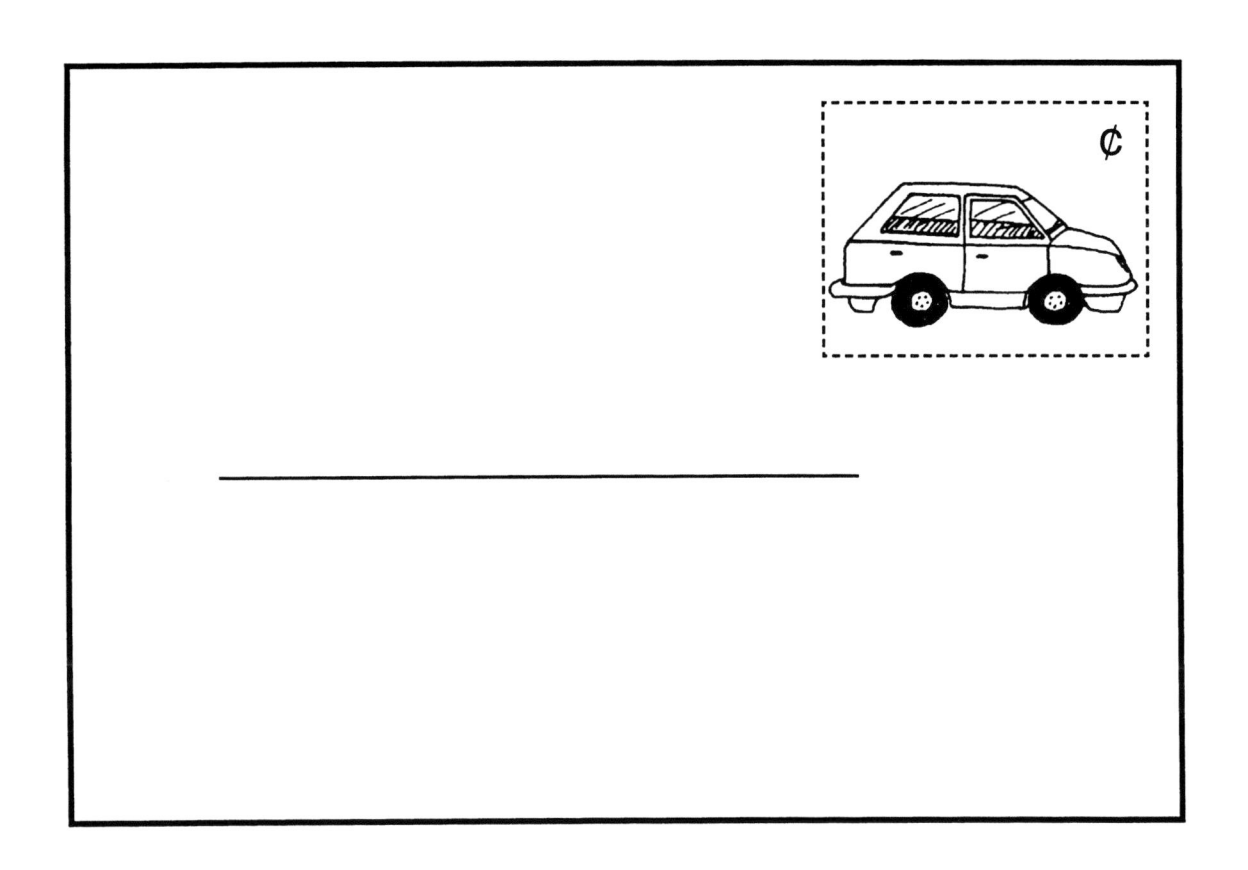

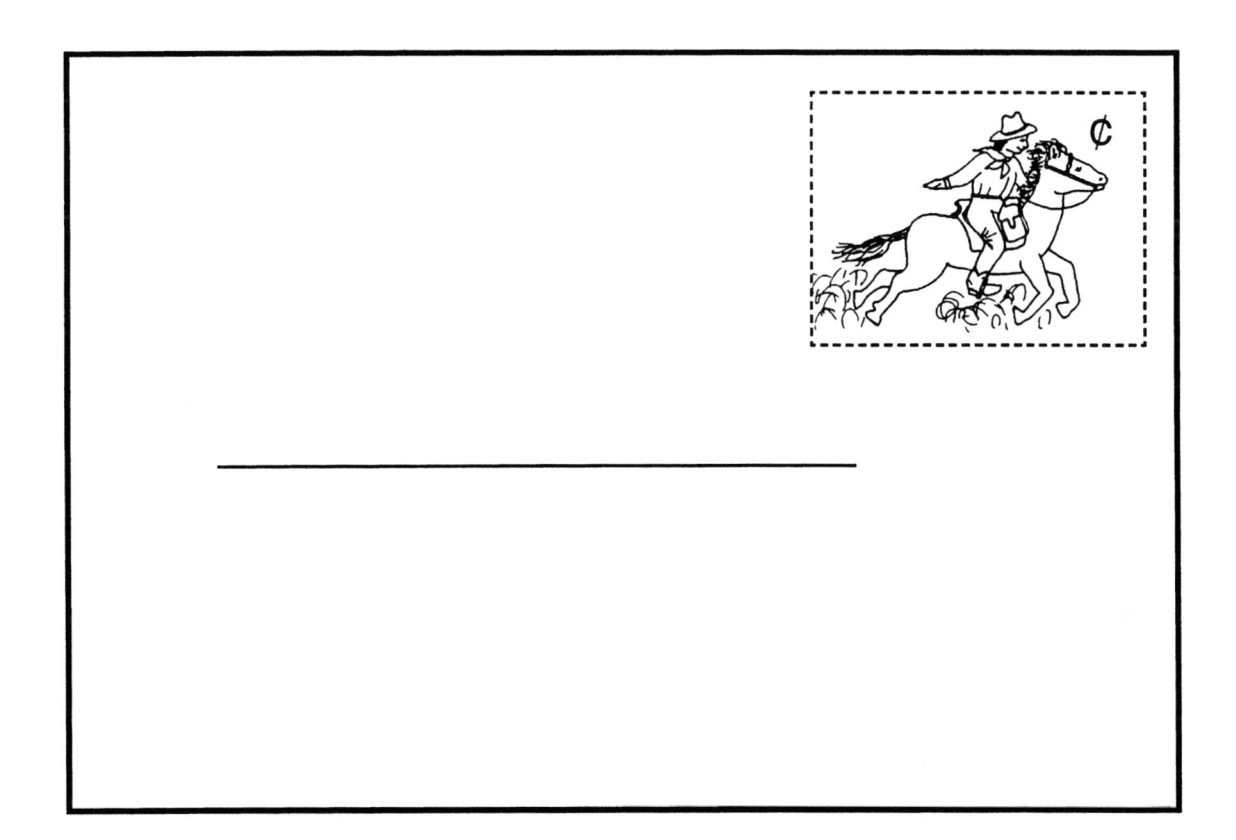

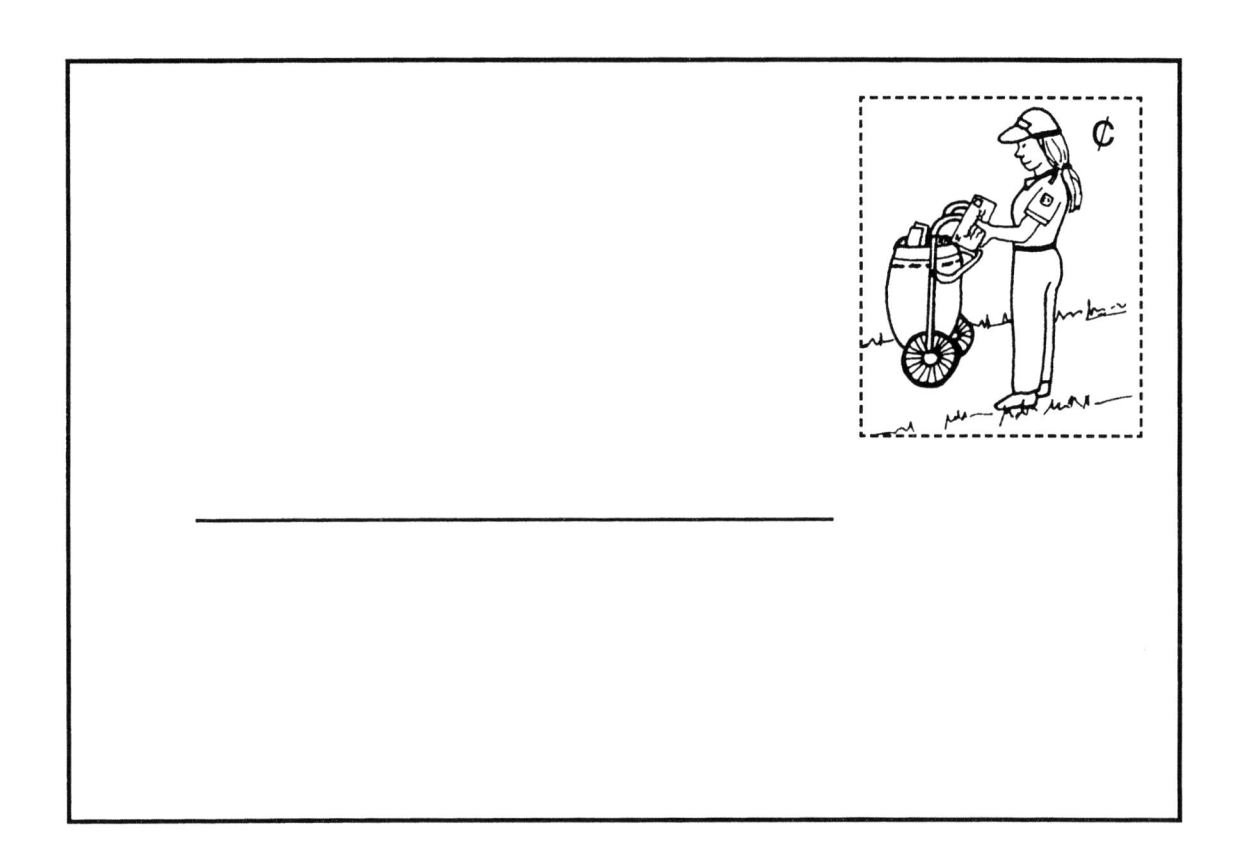

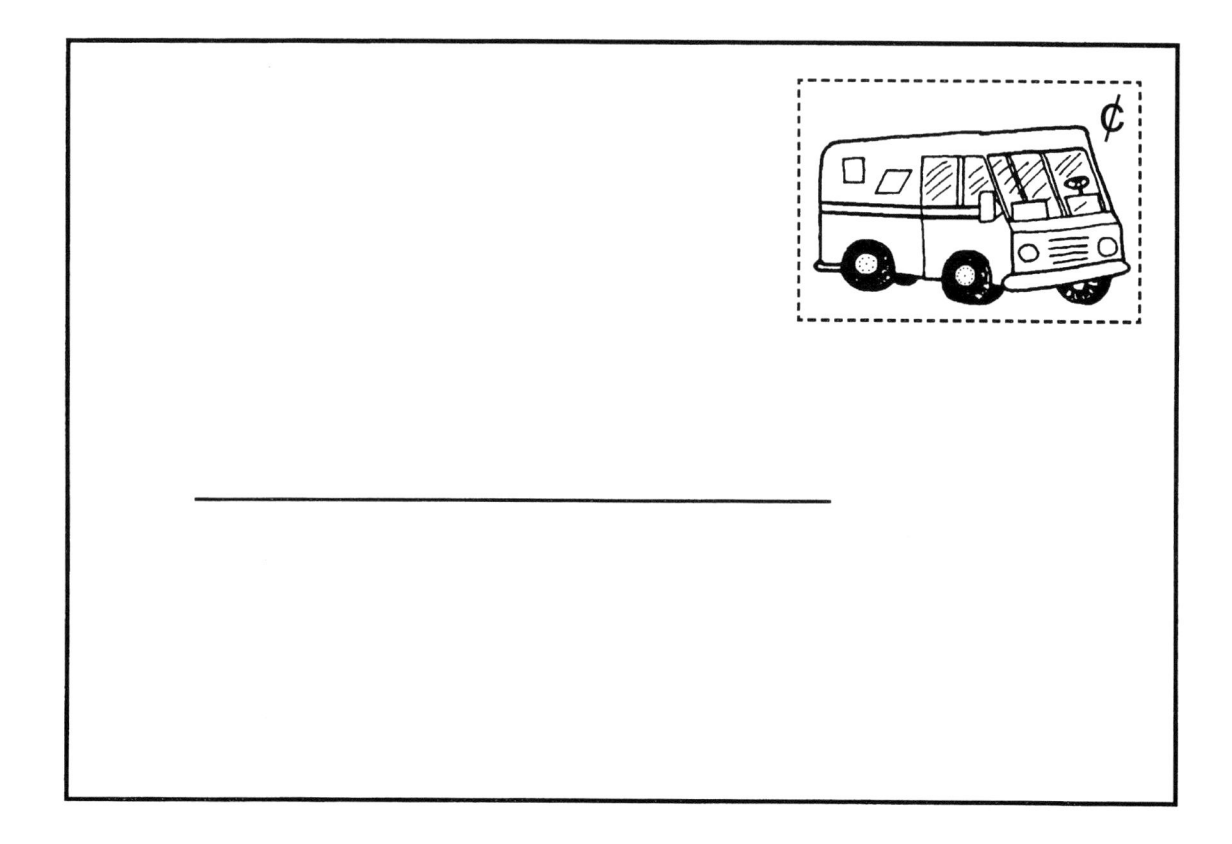

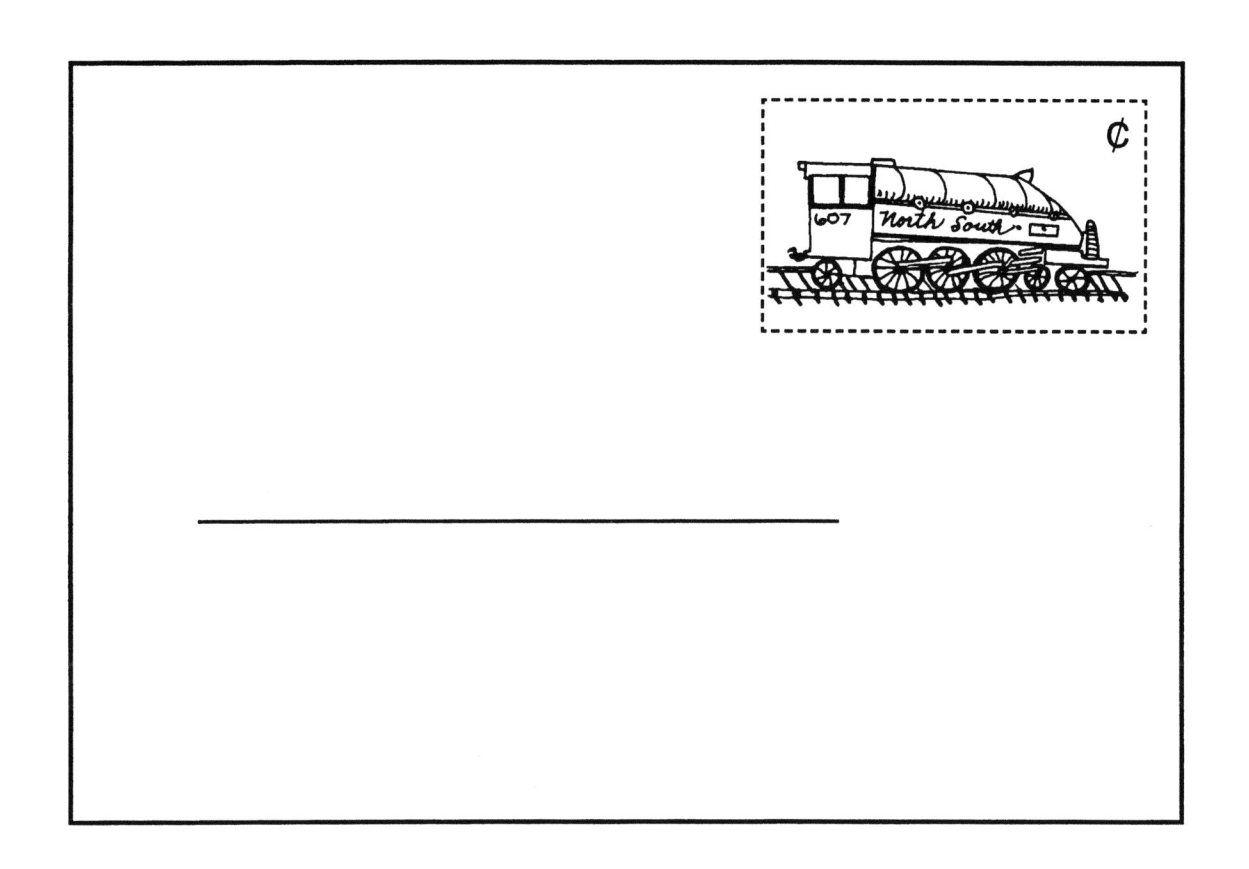

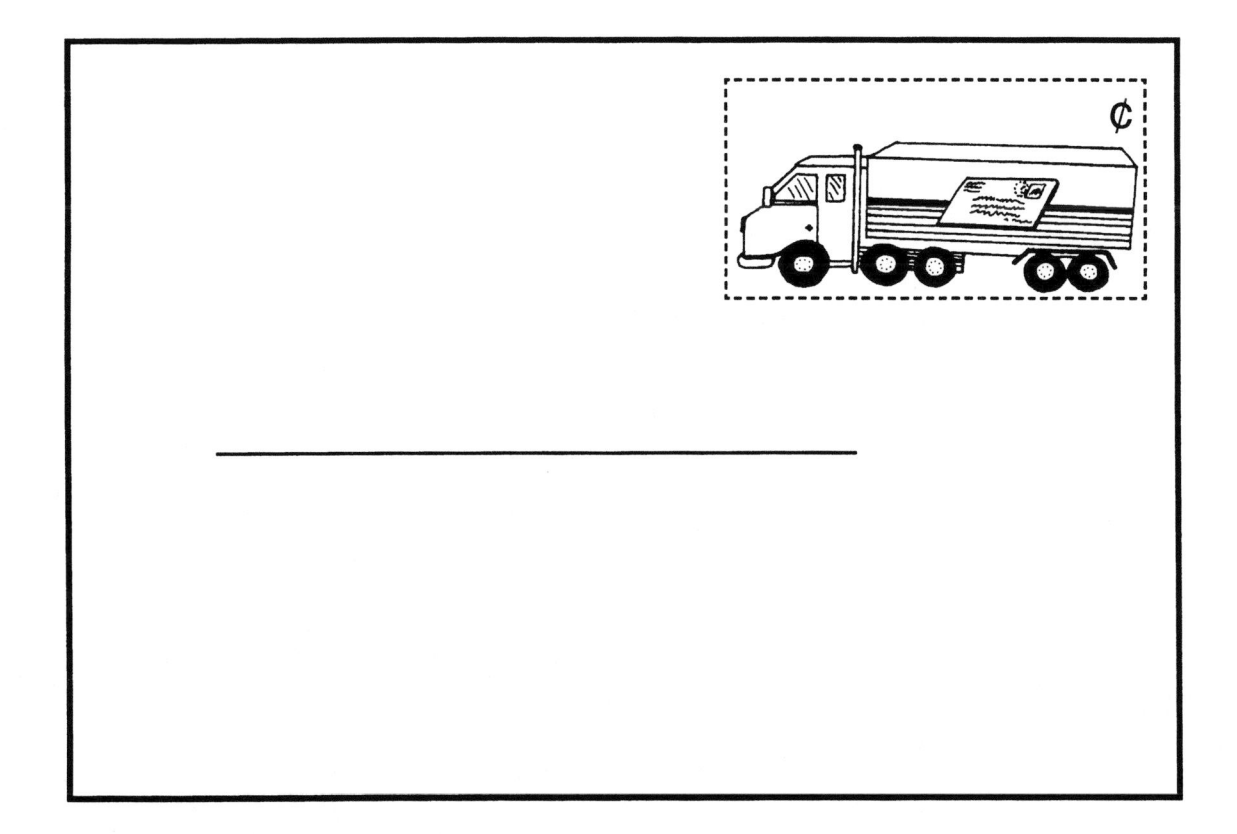

Secret Word
Floor Grid Game

Purpose

To differentiate directional concepts in two-dimensional and three-dimensional space. To practice following and giving directional instructions in three-dimensional space. To practice reading and spelling skills.

Materials

Masking tape, blank *Secret Word* grid map, page 93, 16 index cards, black marker and a pencil

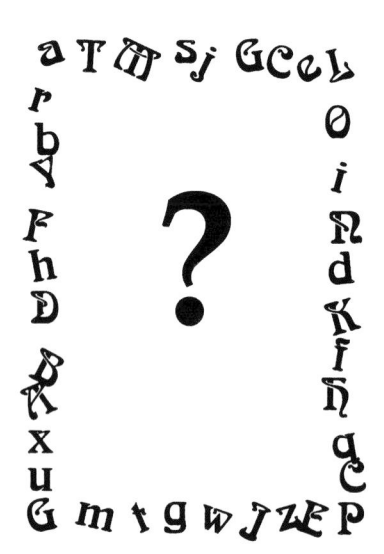

Procedure

- Using the tape, make a floor grid as described on page 104.

- Before starting the game, choose a simple spelling word or vocabulary word at the child's reading level to be the "secret word." Using the blank grid map and pencil, print each letter of the secret word in a grid square. Mix the letters so that they are in a random order. Draw a line from the starting square to the first letter of the word. Next, draw a line from the first letter to the second letter and so on. Remember to draw only vertical and horizonal lines.

- Using the black marker, print each letter of the secret word on an index card. You will have several blank index cards remaining. Next, refer to the grid map to place each index card face down in its corresponding floor grid square. Place the blank index cards in squares without letters so that all 16 floor grid squares have cards. Now you are ready to play the game.

- Tell the child, "There is a secret word hidden in these squares. Each square has a card in it. Some of the cards have letters printed on them. The letters spell the secret word. Your job is to find each letter in correct order. After you have found all of the letters, try to guess the secret word."

- Continue instructing the child by saying, "Stand in the starting square. I will use the *Secret Word* map to direct you to each letter. Listen to my

---

LEVEL 3—ENVIRONMENT AS A REFERENCE POINT

instructions. I may tell you to go forward, backward, left or right. I will also tell you how many squares to move. Remember to stay faced in the same direction as you move. When you get to a square with a letter, I will say, 'pick up.' Pick up the card and turn it over. Is there a letter on it? What is the letter? Keep the letter card to help you guess the secret word."

- Refer to the map to give the child instructions to find each letter of the secret word. When she has collected all of the letter cards, say, "Now put the letters together to spell out a word. What is the secret word?"

Observe

Can the child follow your directional instructions to find each letter of the secret word? Can she orient her body in space correctly? If the child has difficulty orienting in space, use extra visual cues and give additional instructions as follows: "Do you see the clock on the wall? When you are in the grid, make sure that you are always facing the clock. When you need to move right or left, sidestep so that you are always facing the clock." Observe the child's reading skills. Can the child put the letters together to guess the secret word?

More Ideas

Use this activity to build reading skills. When the child finds a letter, ask him to say the letter and its sound out loud.

After the child has guessed the secret word, expand the activity. Ask the child to 1) define the secret word, 2) spell the secret word from memory with eyes closed, 3) print the secret word on the chalkboard and 4) write the secret word in cursive.

Make this activity more challenging by allowing the child to choose the secret word, draw a word map, print each letter on a card, hide the cards in the floor grid and give you forward, backward, left and right instructions to find each letter.

Keep extra index cards and blank grid maps available to repeat the game with several secret words. Save each completed word map and its corresponding letter cards for future use.

Looking for Landmarks

Purpose

To differentiate directional concepts in three-dimensional space. To give and follow directional instructions in three-dimensional space. To develop wayfinding readiness.

Materials

None

Procedure

- Before the game, plan a short walk. You might walk to a building, a playground or a store. Plan a round-trip route so that you start and end at the same place. Make sure to include several direction changes in your route. Now you are ready to begin the game.

- Tell the child, "We are going on a walk. Your job is to look for a landmark every time we make a turn. A landmark is an object that you see along the way. It helps you remember where you are. A landmark can be anything that doesn't move, for example, a tree, a sign or a drinking fountain. I will help you look for landmarks on our walk. Try to remember them in correct order."

- Begin your walk at a starting point. Choose a starting point with a distinctive landmark, such as a flagpole.

- When you are about to turn, stop and help the child choose a landmark. For example, say, "We turn right at the mailbox."

- Continue walking and making turns until you get back to your original starting point. During the walk, pause from time to time to look back at your route and the landmarks you passed along the way.

- After the walk, sit down with the child and review your route from beginning to end. Try to remember each landmark in sequence as well as which direction you turned at each landmark.

LEVEL 3—ENVIRONMENT AS A REFERENCE POINT

Observe

Is the child aware of the environment? Can he focus attention on finding distinctive landmarks along the way? Can he apply directional concepts to the environment? At the end of the walk, can the child recall each landmark in correct sequence? Can the child recall which direction he turned at each landmark?

More Ideas

After the walk, ask the child to draw the route on a piece of paper, including the landmarks.

Go on imaginary walks. Ask the child to imagine a familiar route such as walking at home from the kitchen to the bedroom. Instruct the child to visualize the route and describe landmarks for each turn along the way.

Level 4—Others as a Reference Point

The activities in Level 4 will help children understand that each person views directional concepts from his own perspective. At this level children can easily follow instructions with directional components relative to their own bodies. They can also apply directional concepts to objects and settings in the environment. They are now ready to recognize left and right in people–even when they face in different directions. They will learn to mentally rotate position relative to themselves and project it onto a person facing in the opposite direction. These spatial judgments are made from the point of view of others.

Level 4 skills are necessary for advanced directional tasks. Among these are giving directions to others, dancing with a partner and playing team sports.

The activities in Level 4 focus on the ability to differentiate directional concepts on others and to give directional instructions to others.

Please note that some of the activities in this level are modified from Level 3 activities. Modifying previous activities allows reinforcement through repetition, but at a higher level of challenge.

Paper People Cutouts

Purpose

To differentiate directional concepts on others. To practice visual-motor control and dexterity.

Materials

Reproducible *Paper People* sheets found on pages 146-157, scissors, colored pencils and glue

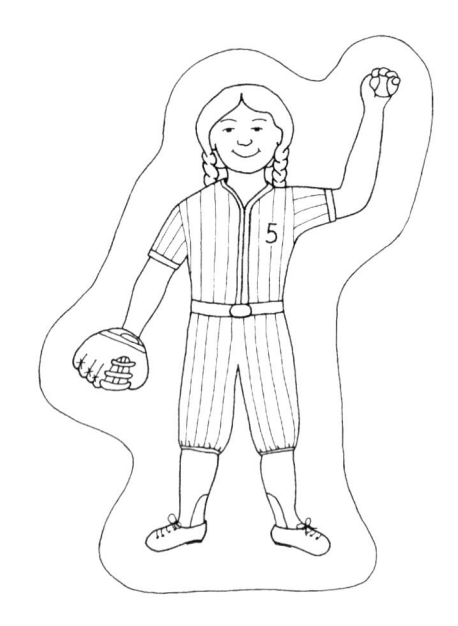

Procedure

- Photocopy the *Paper People* sheets. There are seven paper people to choose from: a Paramedic, a Cheerleader, a Chef, a Baseball Player, a Crossing Guard and a Painter. Each paper person has a front and a back sheet.

- Tell the child, "These are paper people. They are holding different things to help them do their jobs. Each person has a front and a back."

- Continue instructing the child by saying, "Your job is to cut out the front and back of a paper person. Try to cut along the outside line."

- After the child has cut out the front and back, say, "Now glue the front and back together. Make sure that the body parts line up correctly. When you are finished, you may color both sides of your paper person."

- Discuss the completed cutout with the child. Tell the child, "Hold your paper person so that you are looking at the back. What is the right arm doing? What is the left arm doing?"

- Continue instructing the child by saying, "Now turn your paper person over so that you are looking at the front. Do you see the person's face? Where do you see the person's right arm now? Where is the left arm?"

- Ask the child, "How does the front of the cutout compare with the back of the cutout? What happens to left and right when you turn the cutout over?"

LEVEL 4—OTHERS AS A REFERENCE POINT

Observe

Is the child able to differentiate left and right on the cutout? Does he understand left and right from the perspectives of front and back?

More Ideas

Ask the child to pose like the paper person.

Use the paper person cutouts to discuss career themes.

Paramedic

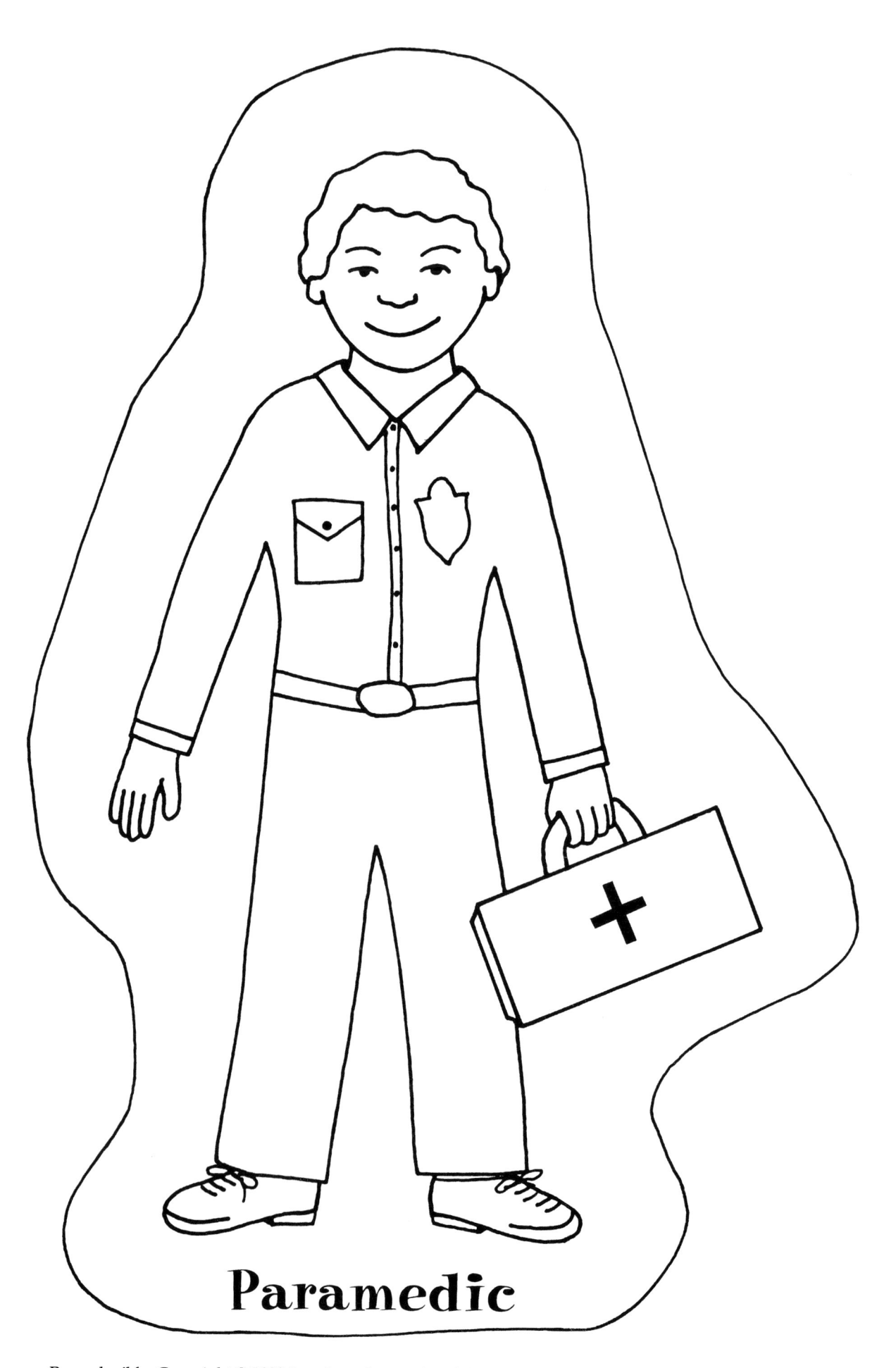

147

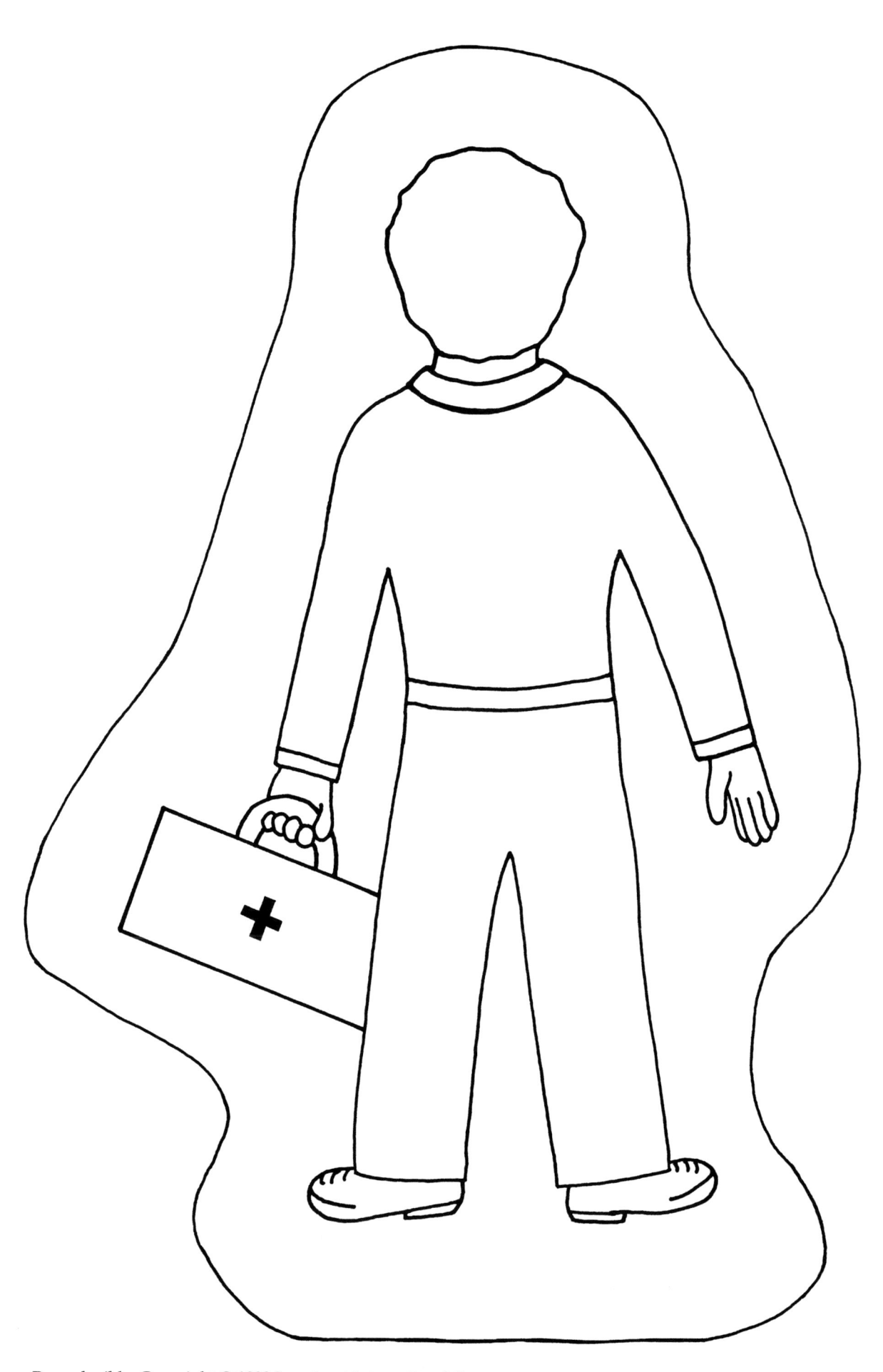

Cheerleader

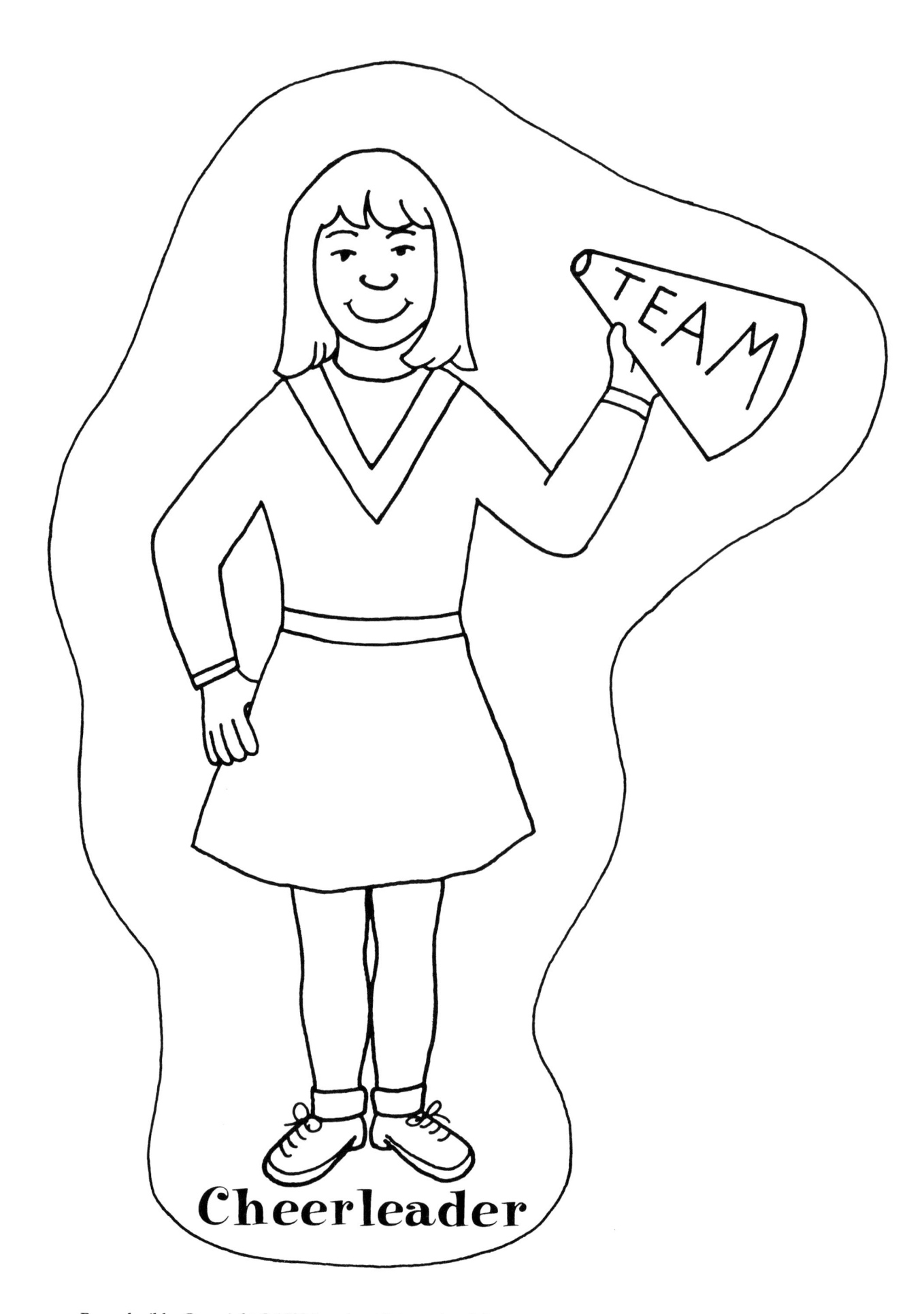

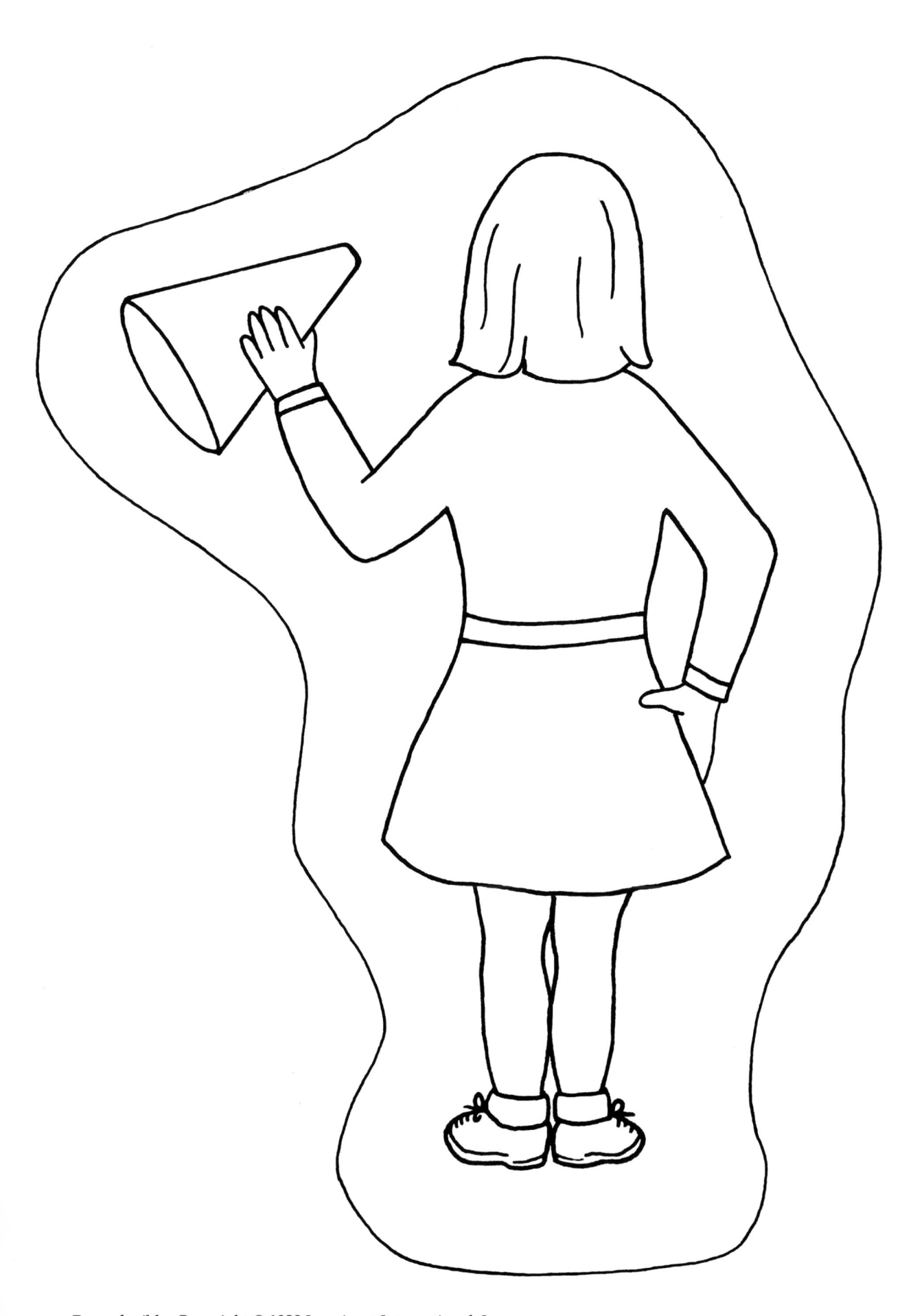

Reproducible. Copyright © 1999 Imaginart International, Inc.

149

Chef

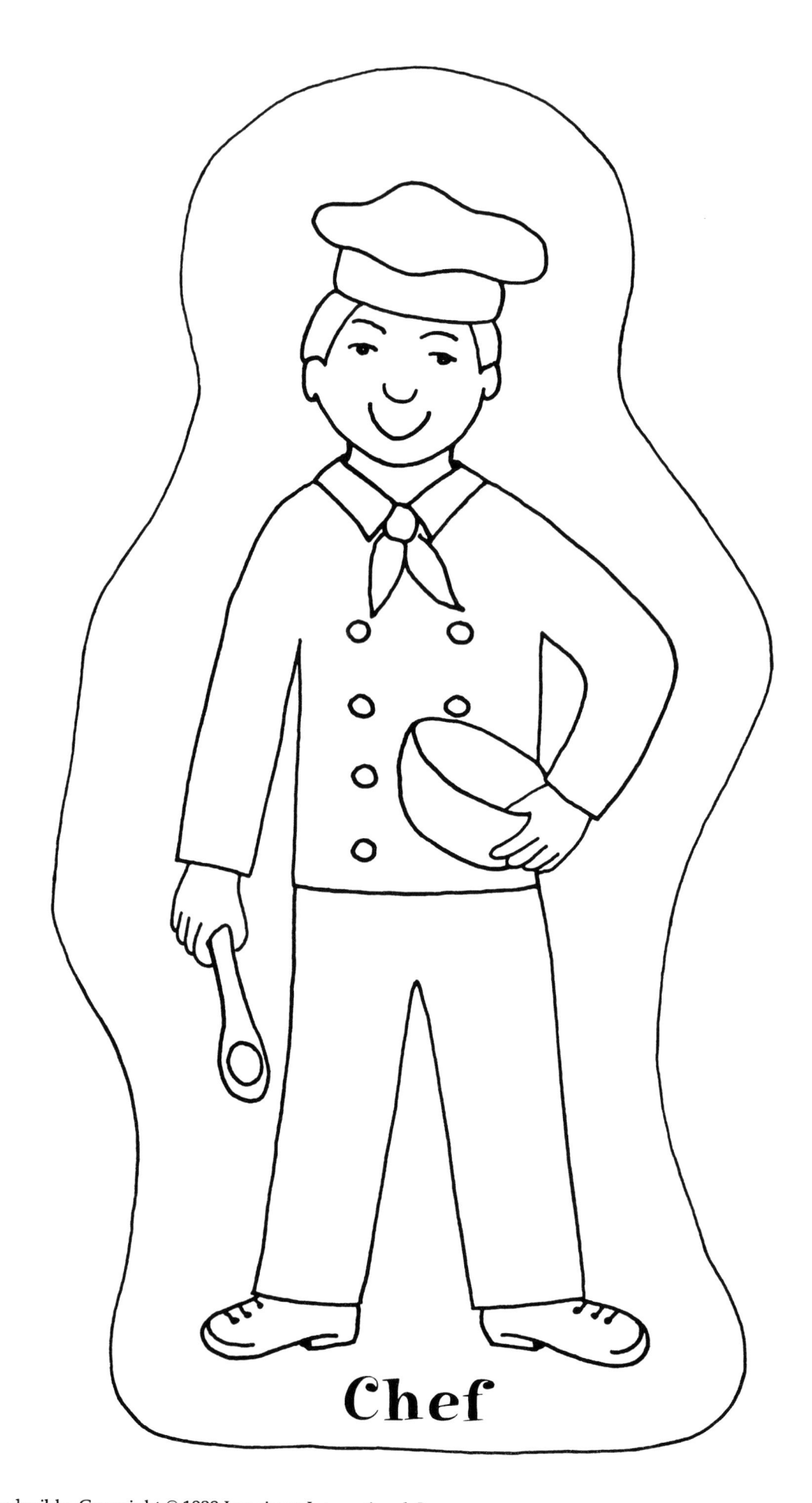

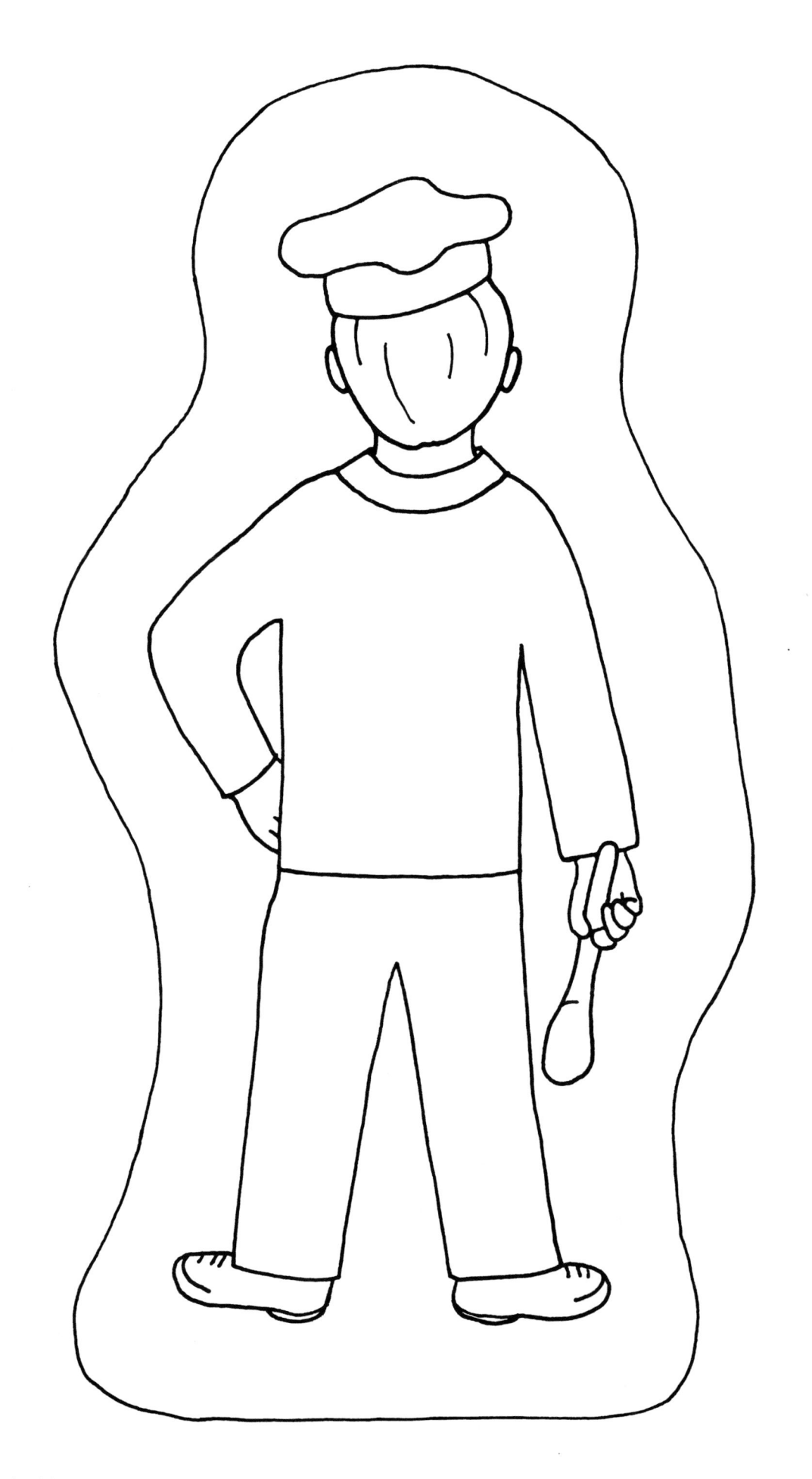

Baseball Player

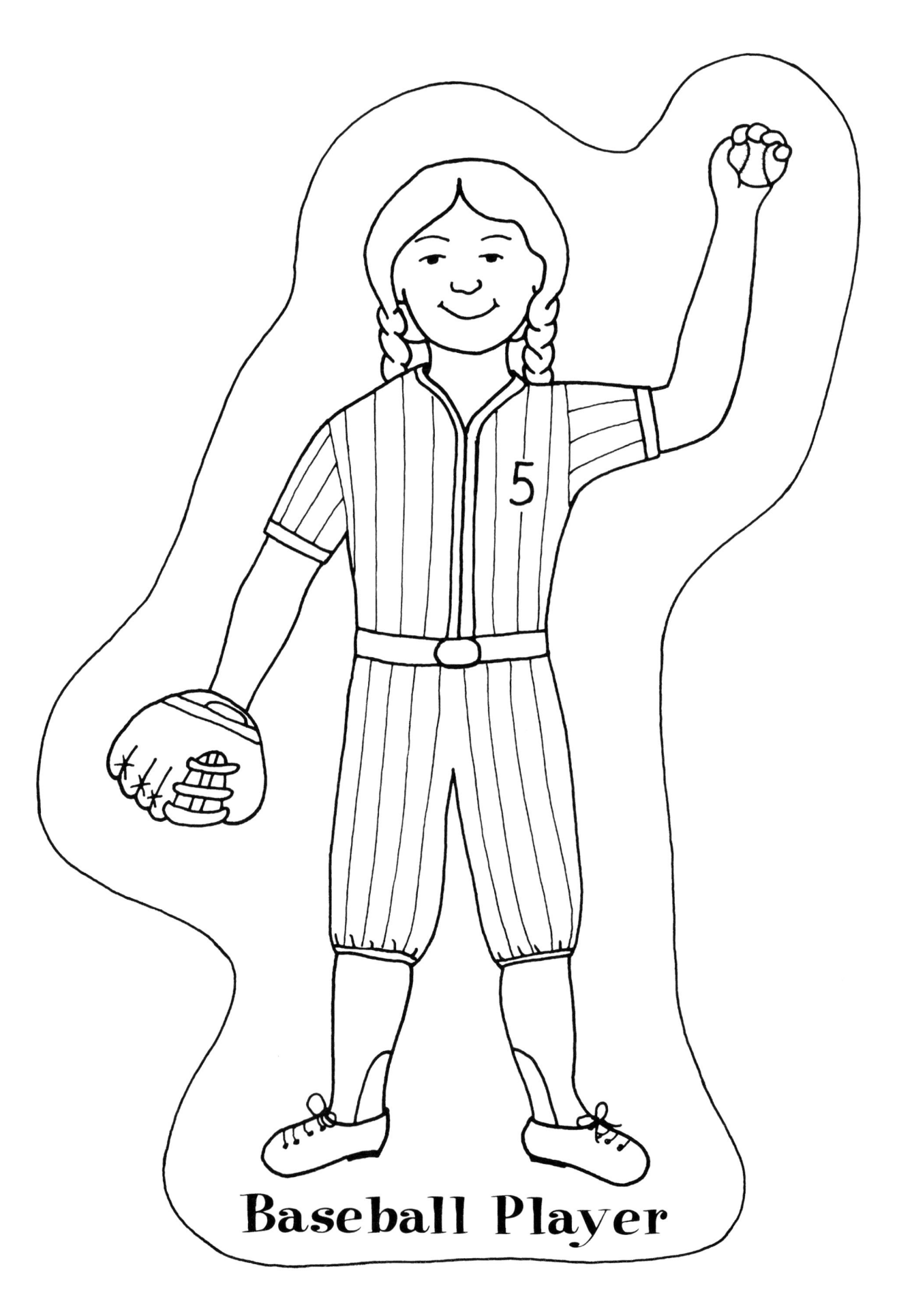

Reproducible. Copyright © 1999 Imaginart International, Inc.

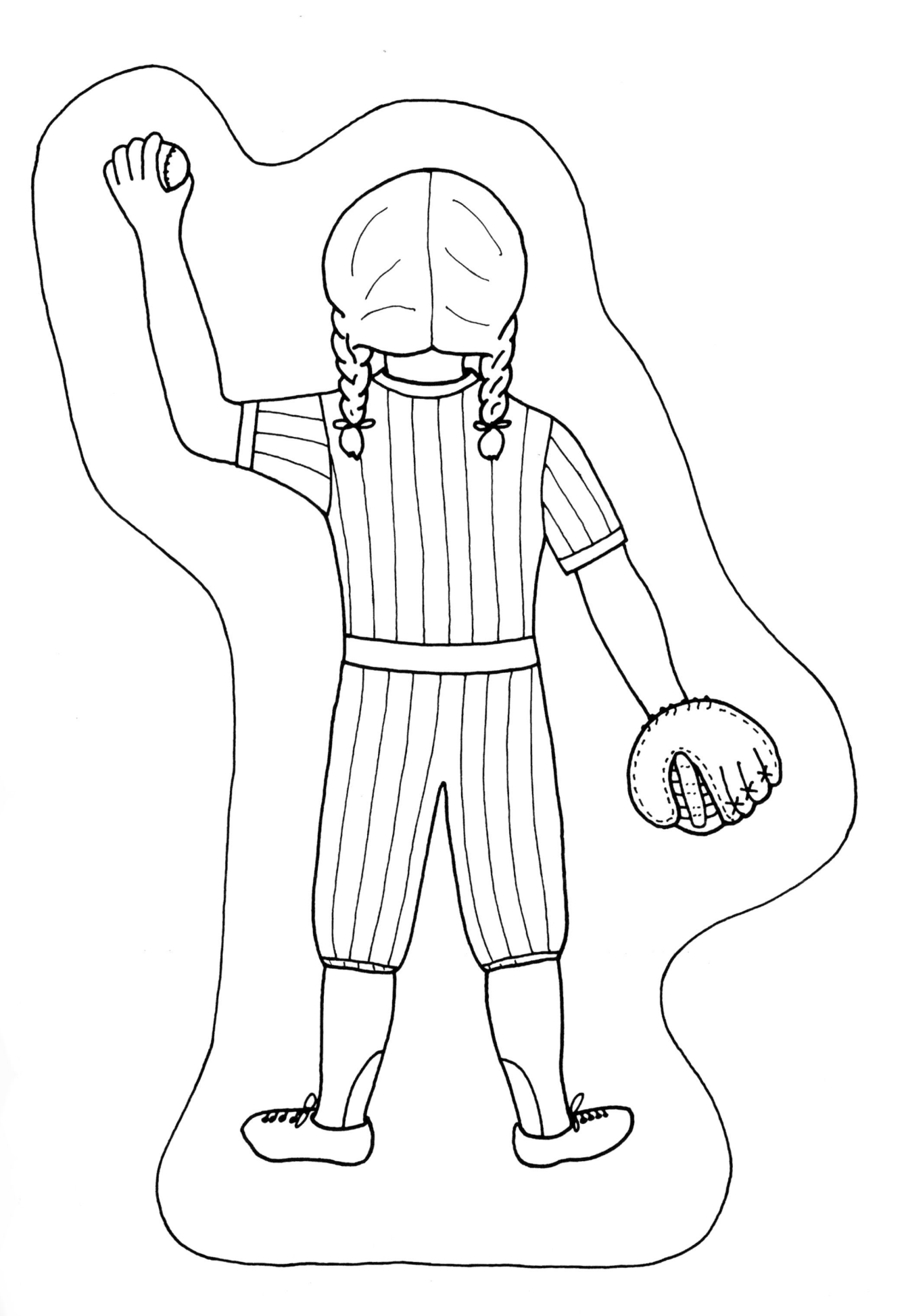

Reproducible. Copyright © 1999 Imaginart International, Inc.

STOP

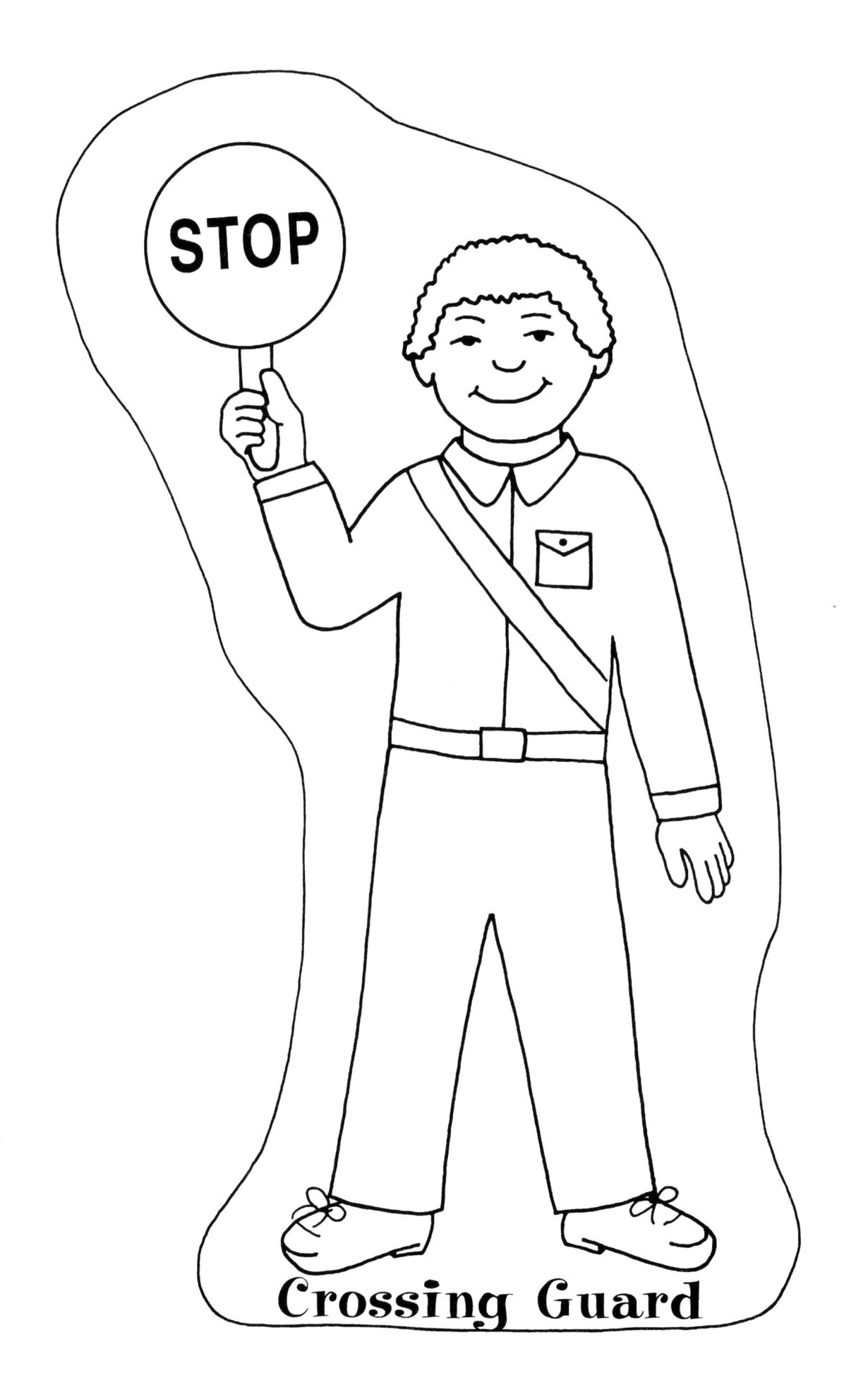

Crossing Guard

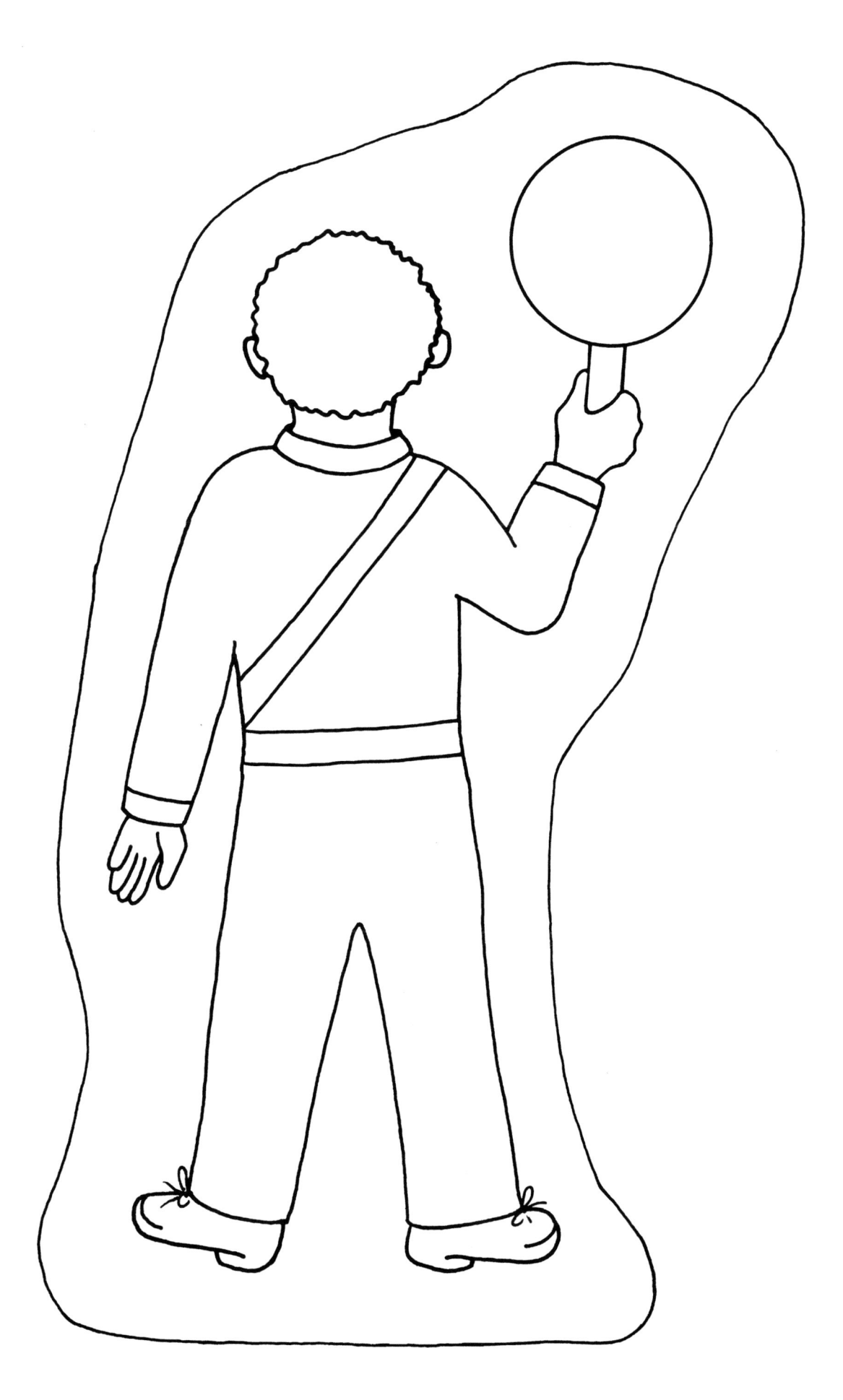

Reproducible. Copyright © 1999 Imaginart International, Inc.

Painter

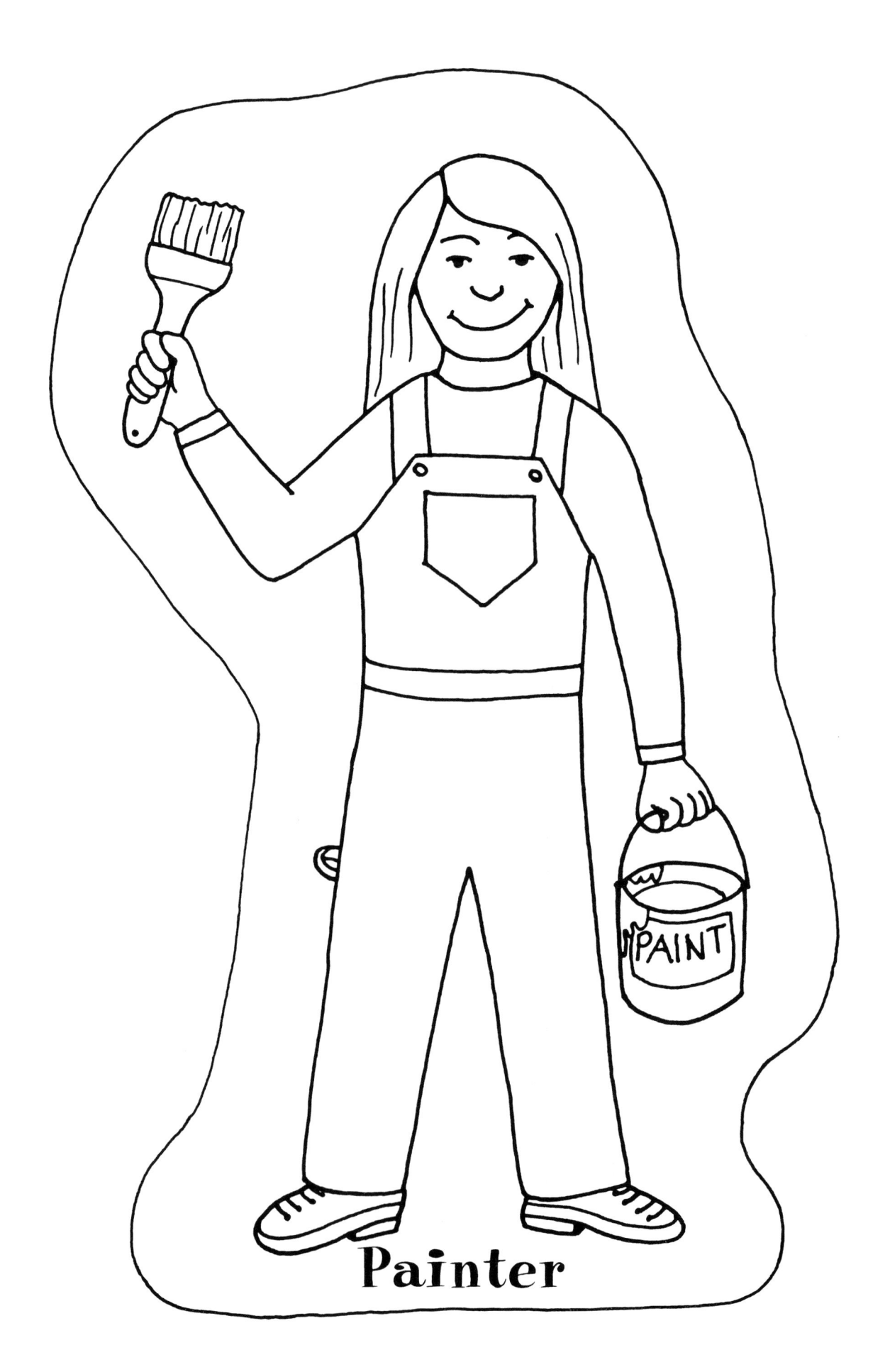

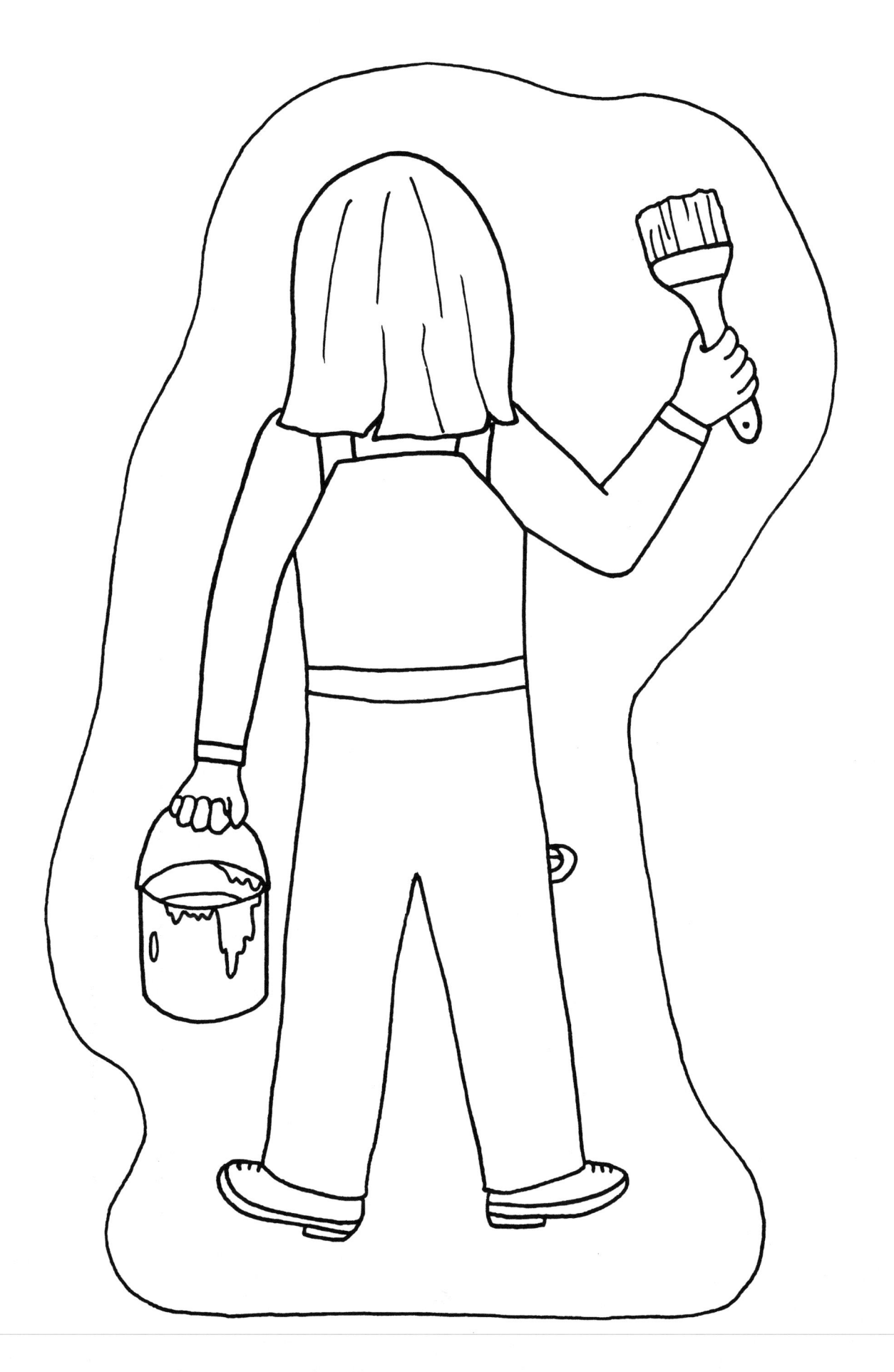

Picture Poses

Purpose

To differentiate directional concepts on others. To reinforce body awareness and motor planning through imitation of postures.

Materials

Set of 8 reproducible *Picture Poses* found on pages 160-167

Procedure

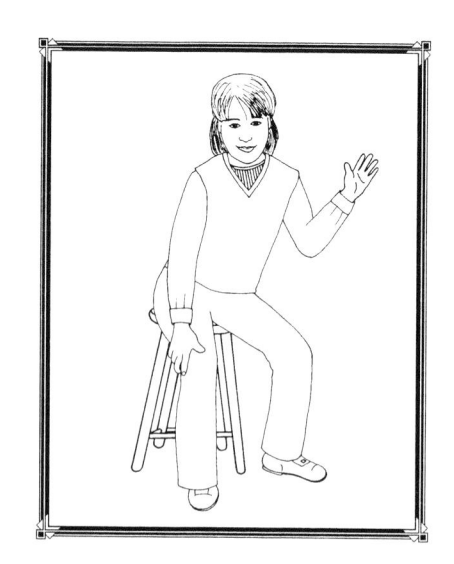

- Photocopy the *Picture Poses*. If you wish, attach each picture to tagboard and laminate for durability.

- Show the child the *Picture Poses* and say, "Pretend that you are a photographer. If you were taking pictures of these people, you would be facing them. Remember that when you are facing someone, their left and right is the reverse or opposite of yours."

- Hold up the *Picture Poses* one at a time and say, "I will point to a left or right body part on the picture. Tell me if the body part that I am pointing to is left or right. Remember to give your answer from the point of view of the person in the picture."

- After the child has demonstrated mastery of the concept by identifying left and right body parts correctly, continue the game by saying, "Now choose one of the *Picture Poses*. Try to imitate the person in the picture by posing in the same position. Make sure that your left and right body parts match the picture. I will pretend to be the photographer and take a picture of you."

- Ask the child to hold the pose and describe the position of their left and right body parts. For example, "My right hand is on my right knee." Then pretend to take a picture of the child.

LEVEL 4—OTHERS AS A REFERENCE POINT

Observe

Can the child identify left and right body parts on the picture accurately? Can she imitate the picture pose correctly?

More Ideas

Allow the child to make up a pose.

Take real pictures of people in various poses. You might use the child's friends or classmates.

Allow the child to be the photographer who tells the person how to pose.

Cut out pictures of people in various poses from magazines to discuss.

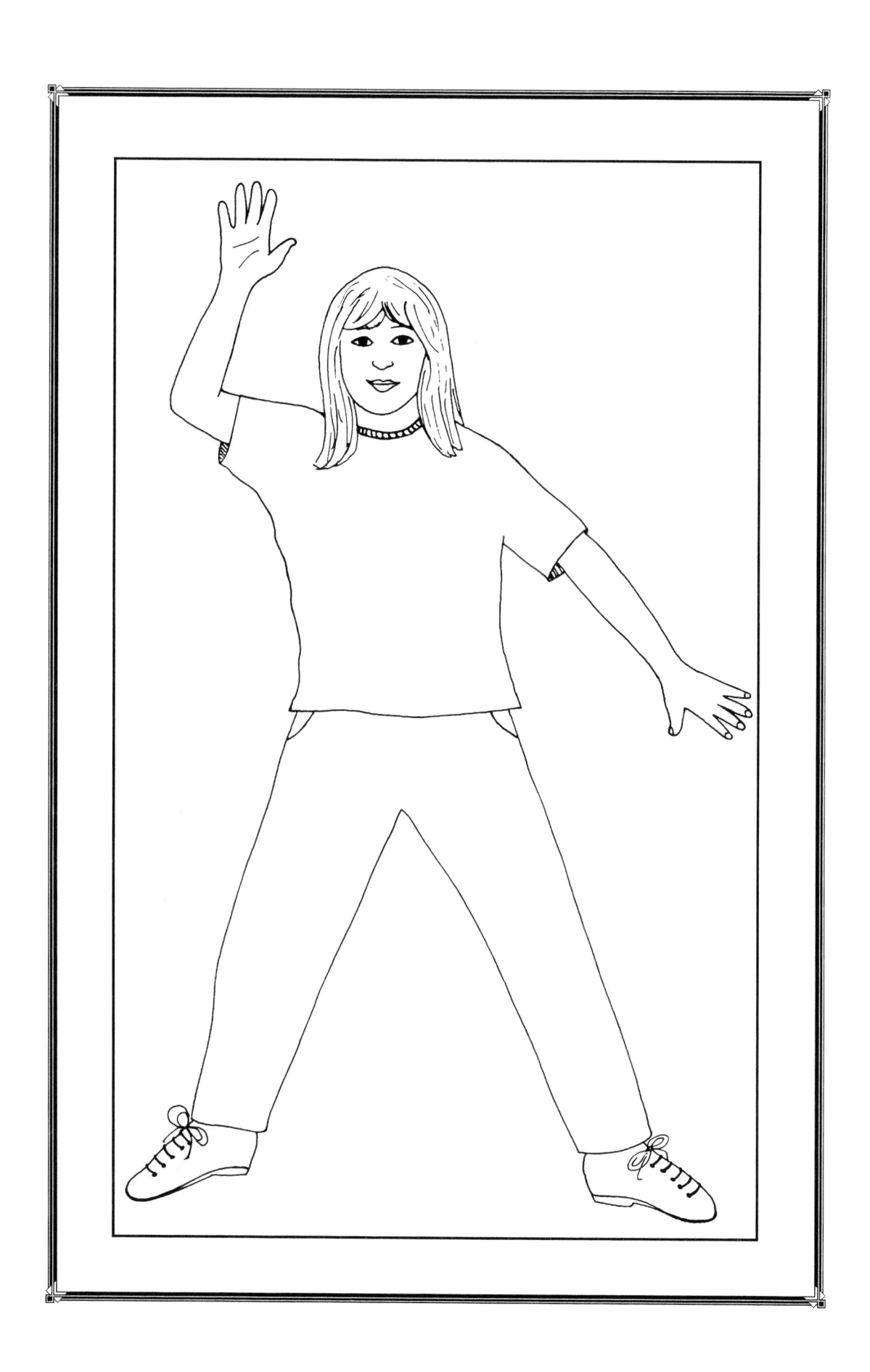

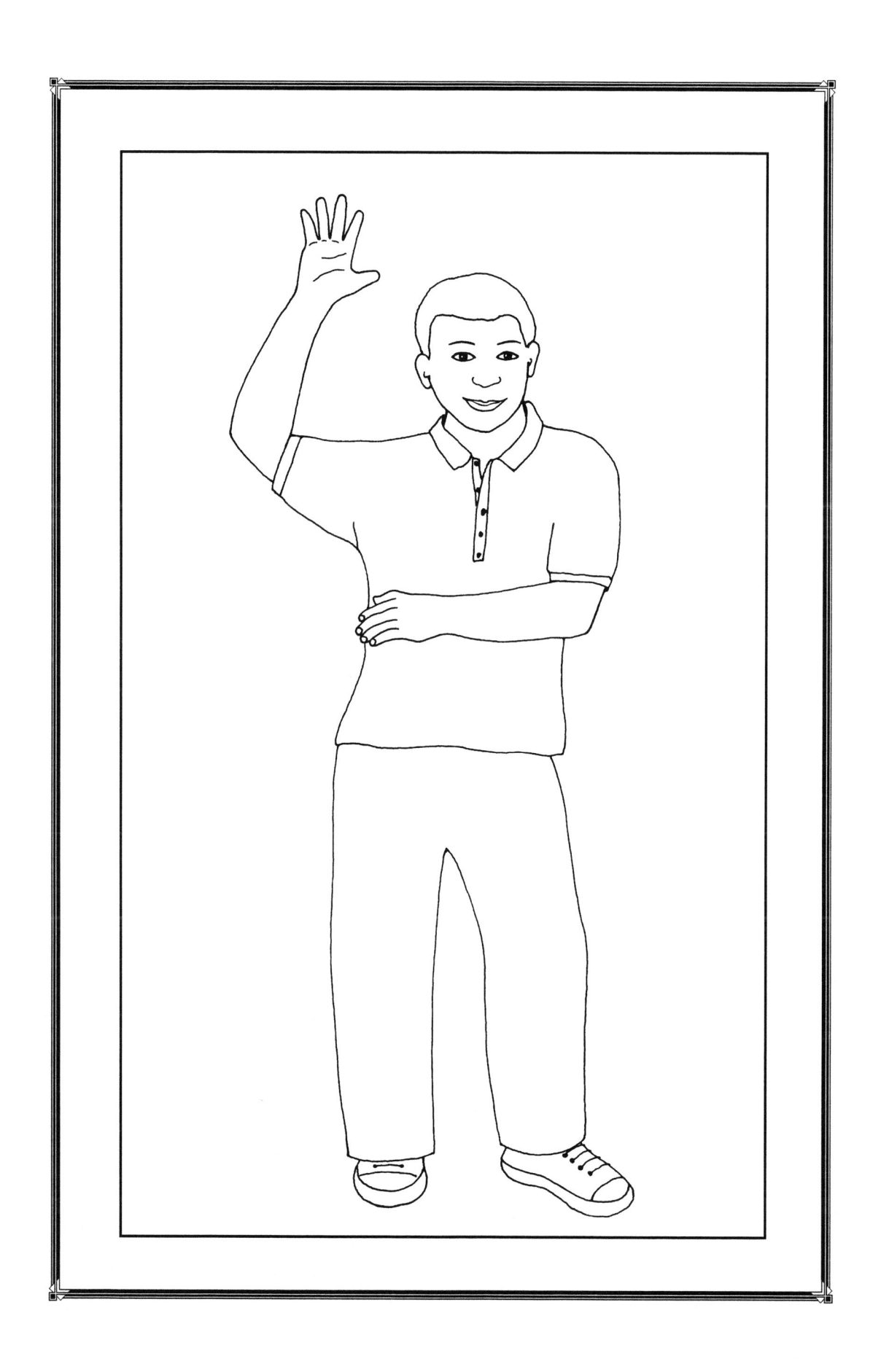

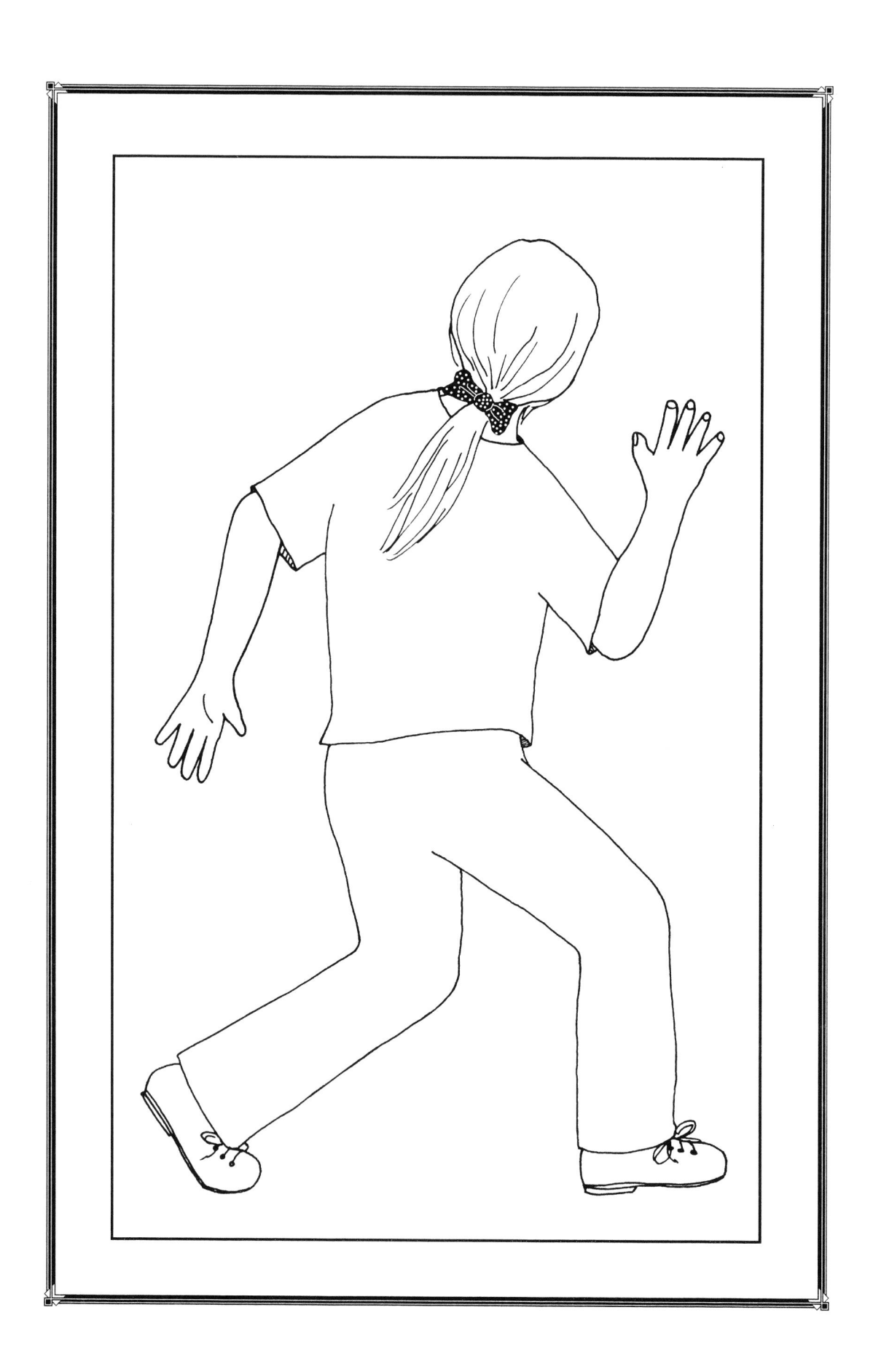

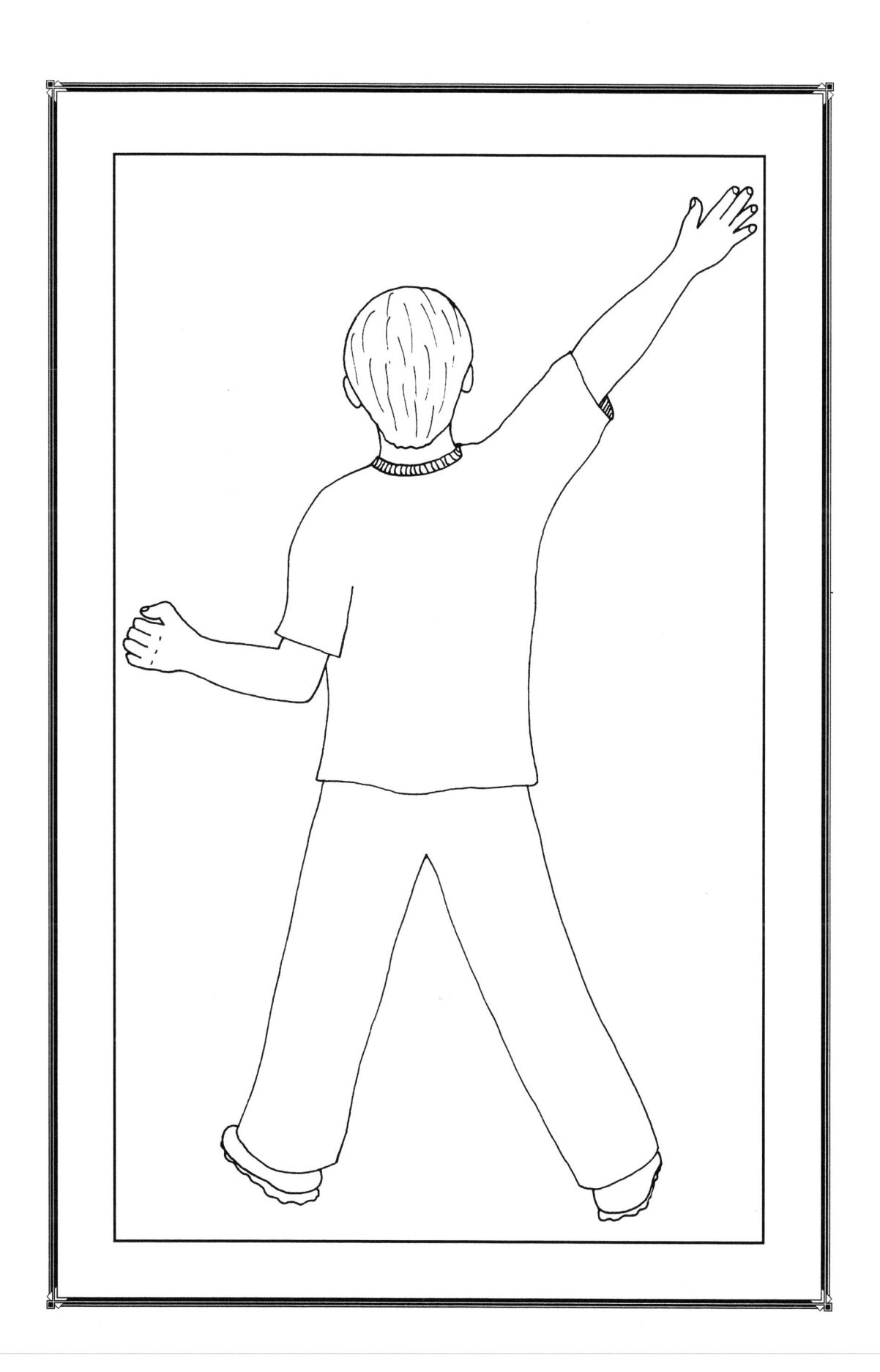

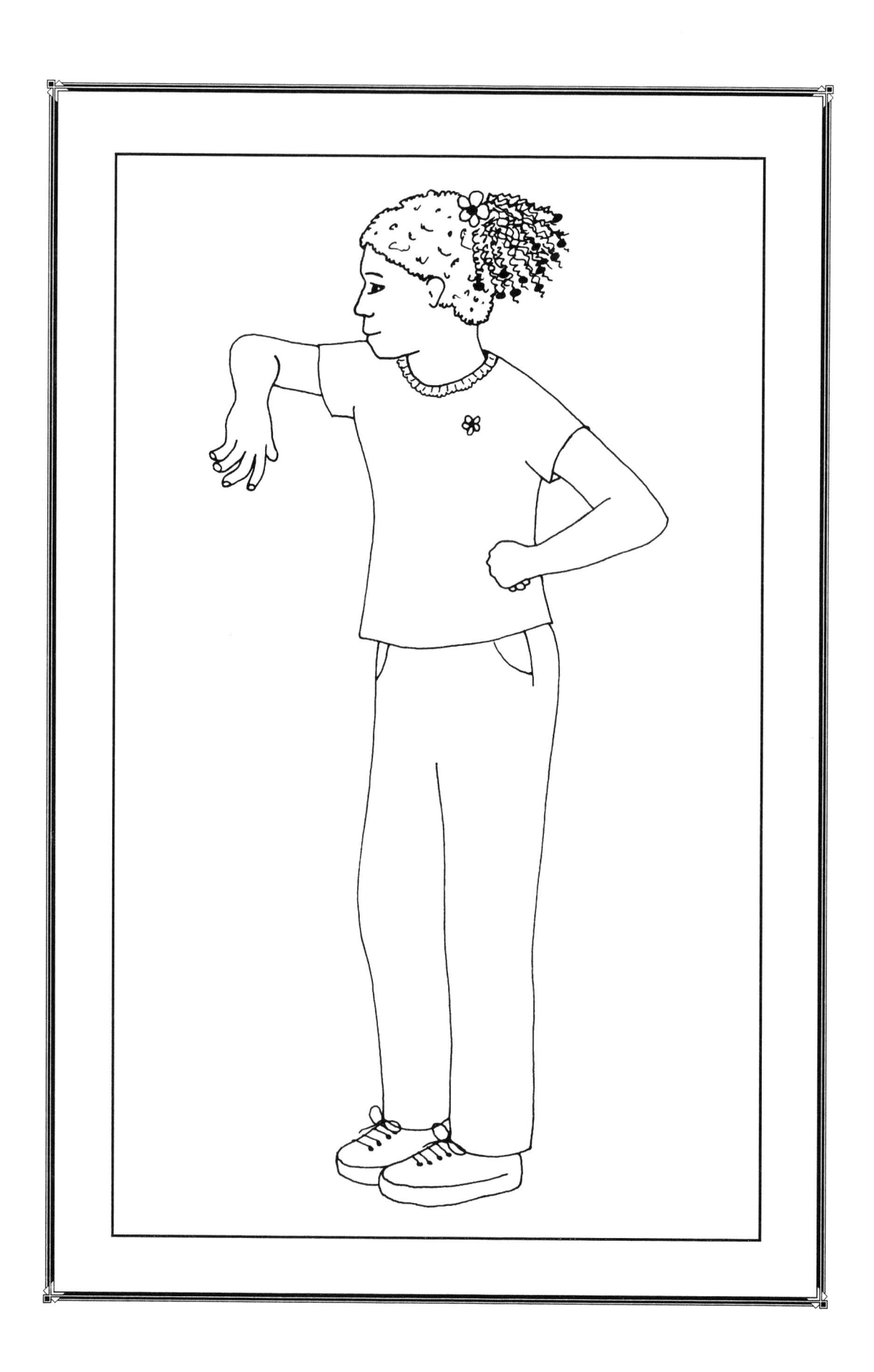

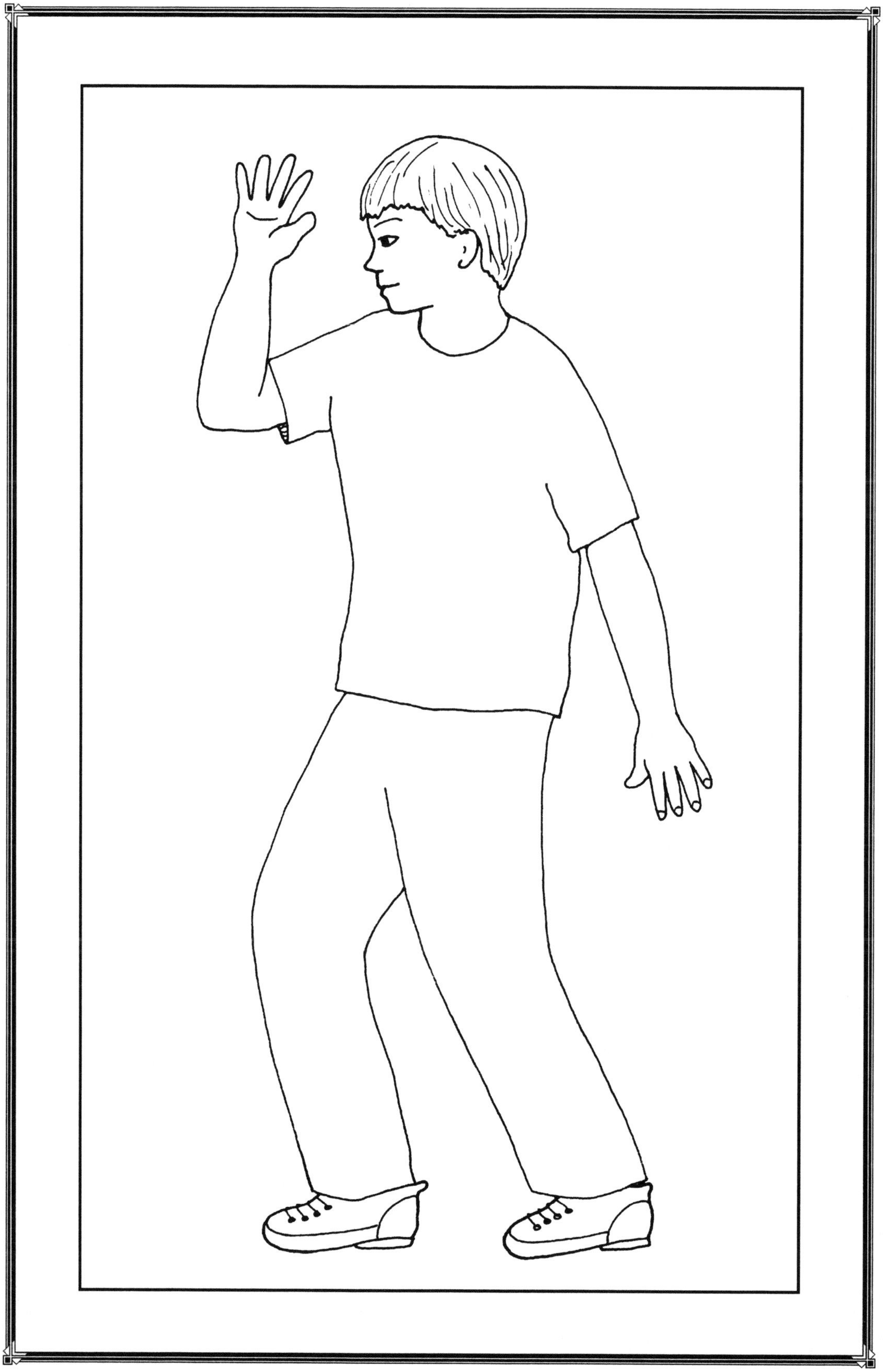

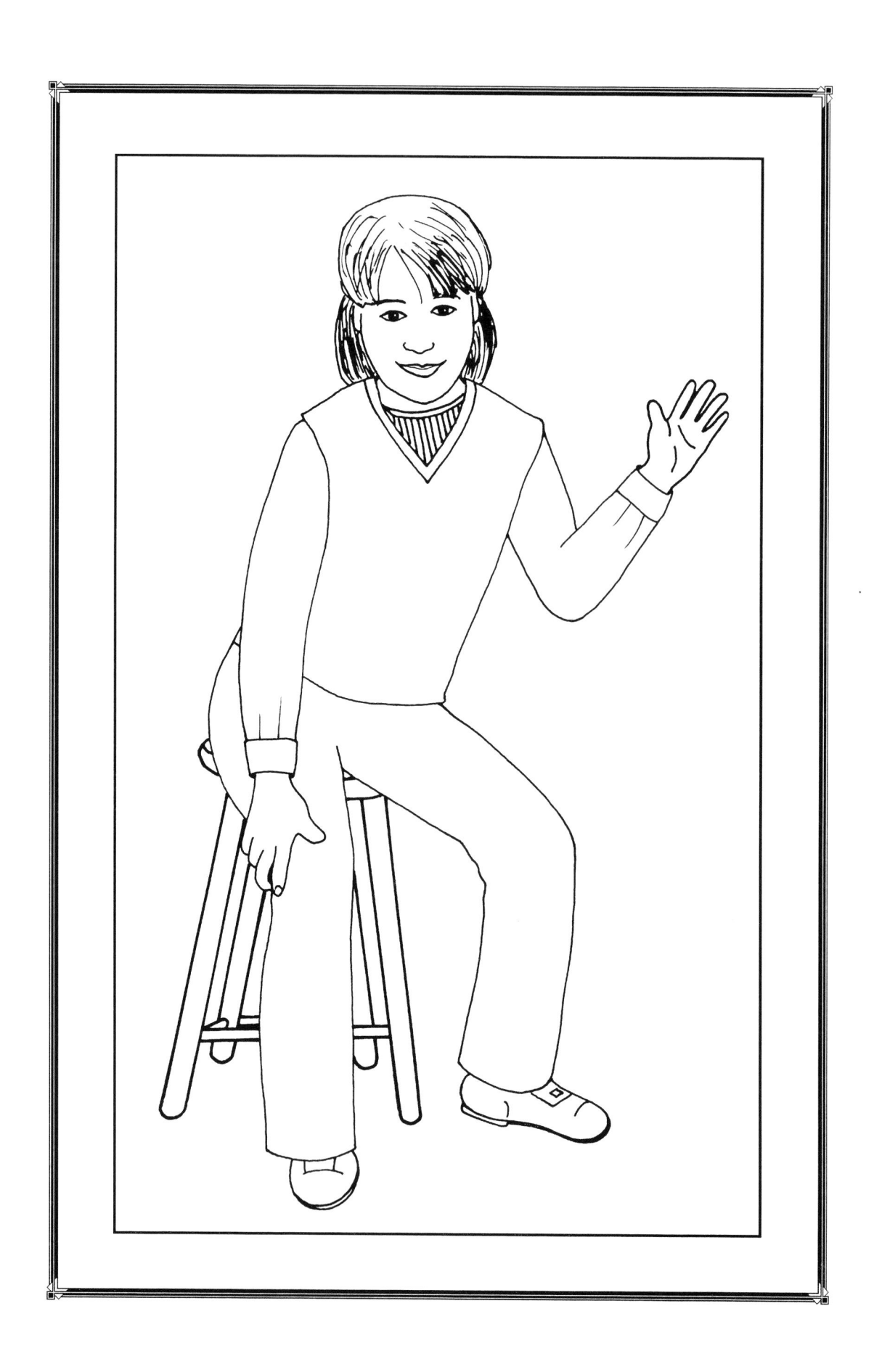

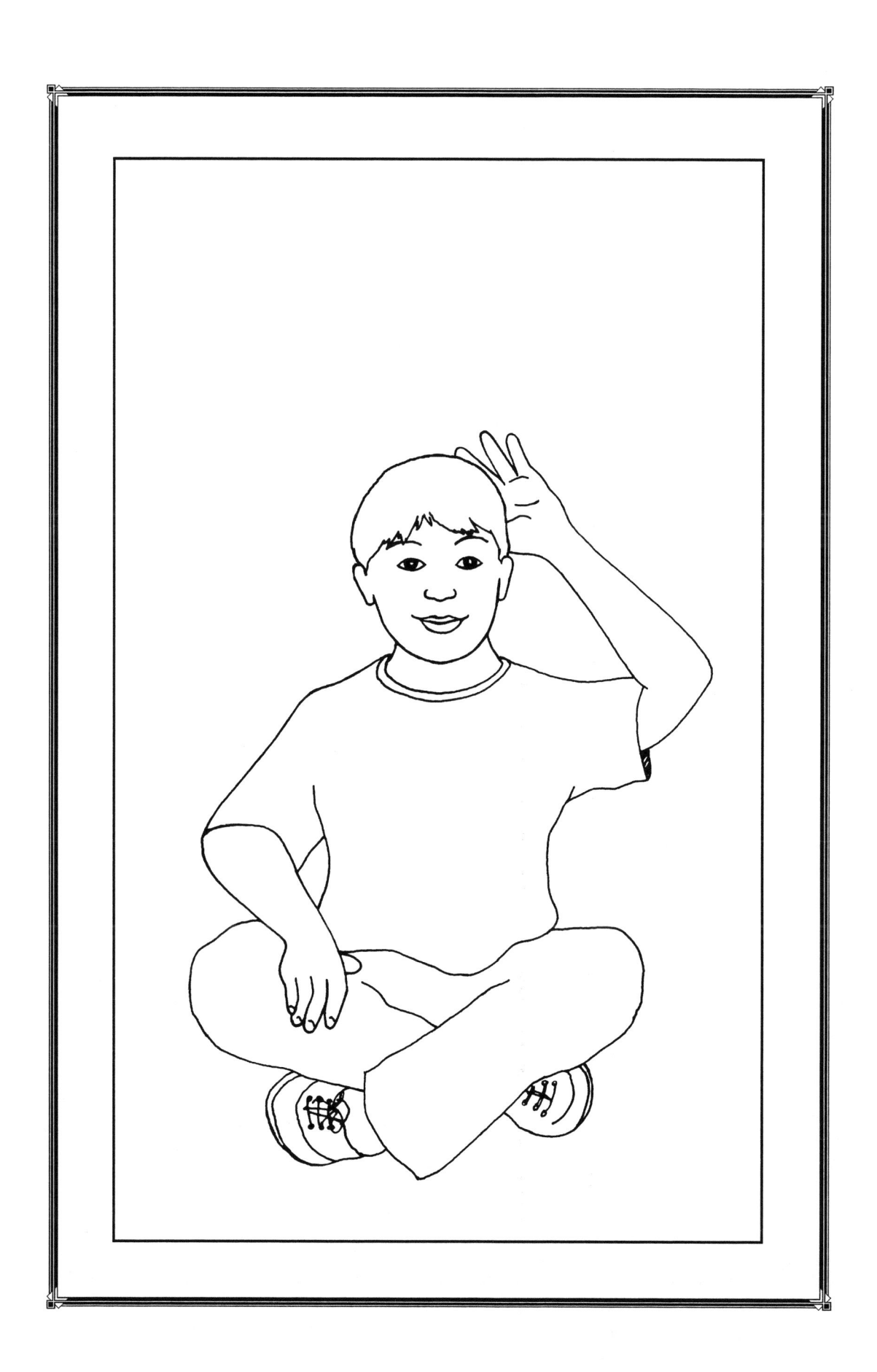

Reproducible. Copyright © 1999 Imaginart International, Inc.

Statue Maker

Purpose

To differentiate directional concepts on others. To reinforce body awareness and motor planning though imitation of postures.

Materials

Set of 8 reproducible *Picture Poses* found on pages 160-167

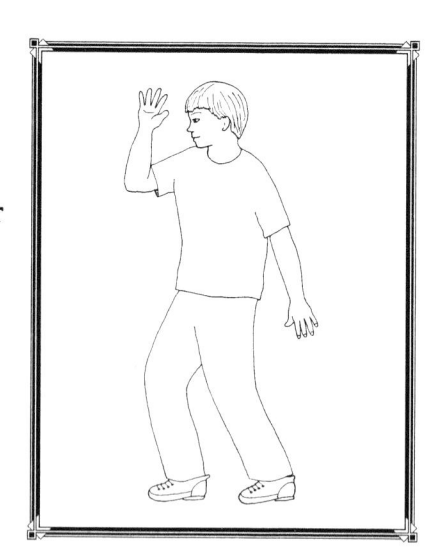

Procedure

- Photocopy the set of *Picture Poses*. If you wish, attach each picture to tagboard and laminate for durability.

- Show the child the *Picture Poses* and say, "I will pretend that I am a Statue Maker. I want to make statues that look like these pictures."

- Discuss each picture pose by saying, "When you look at the picture you are facing it. Remember that when you are facing someone, their left and right is the opposite of yours. I will point to a left or right body part on the picture. Tell me if the body part that I am pointing to is left or right. Remember to give your answer from the point of view of the person in the picture." Now you are ready to play the game.

- Turn all of the pictures face down on the floor and mix them up.

- Continue instructing the child by saying, "Choose one of the pictures and turn it over. Study the pose in the picture and try to remember it. Then turn the picture face down again."

- Tell the child, "Now I will turn you into a statue. Stand up and hold onto my hands. Pretend that you are soft clay. I will spin you around three times. Then I will let go of your hands. When I let go, freeze like a statue. Pose just like the person in your picture. Do you think you can remember the pose?"

- When the child poses say, "Hold your pose while I compare your body position with the picture. Do you think they will match?"

LEVEL 4—OTHERS AS A REFERENCE POINT

Observe

Can the child identify left and right body parts on the picture accurately? Can she recall and imitate the picture pose correctly? Does she have adequate postural control to hold the pose?

More Ideas

Allow the child to make up a unique pose and describe it.

Combine this activity with an art unit. Allow the child to make clay statues of people in different poses.

Design a Pocket T-Shirt

Purpose

To differentiate directional concepts from different positions. To practice visual-motor skills.

Materials

Reproducible *Design a Pocket T-Shirt* sheet found on page 172, scissors and colored pencils

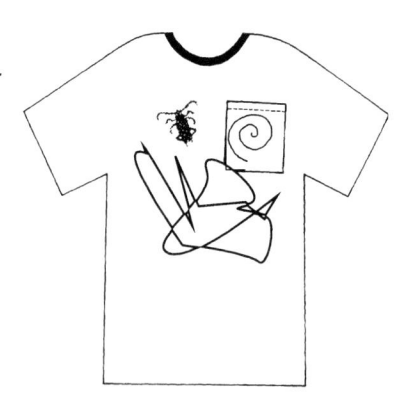

Procedure

- Photocopy the *Design a Pocket T-Shirt* sheet.

- Show the child the *Design a Pocket T-Shirt* sheet saying, "Fashion designers always draw their ideas on paper before making real clothes. Your job is to design your own T-shirt on this paper."

- Continue instructing the child by saying, "Use your scissors to cut out the T-shirt. Try to cut along the thick black line."

- When the T-shirt is cut out, allow the child to decorate both the front and back with markers or crayons. Tell the child, "Remember that the T-shirt has a front and a back. The pocket is on the front. Use your markers or crayons to decorate the T-shirt. You may draw designs, shapes, numbers, flowers—anything that you would like on your T-shirt."

- After the child has decorated the front and back of the pocket T-shirt, discuss directional concepts from different positions. Tell the child, "Look at the front of your T-shirt. Do you see the pocket? Which side of the shirt is the pocket on—the left side or the right side? Now pick up your T-shirt and hold it on your body as if you were wearing it. Now which side is the pocket on—the left side or the right side?"

Observe

Does the child understand that directional concepts can change when viewed from different positions?

LEVEL 4—OTHERS AS A REFERENCE POINT

More Ideas

Use a large sheet of paper to draw a life-sized pocket T-shirt. Cut and decorate as described above.

Allow the child to transfer his design onto a real pocket T-shirt with fabric paint.

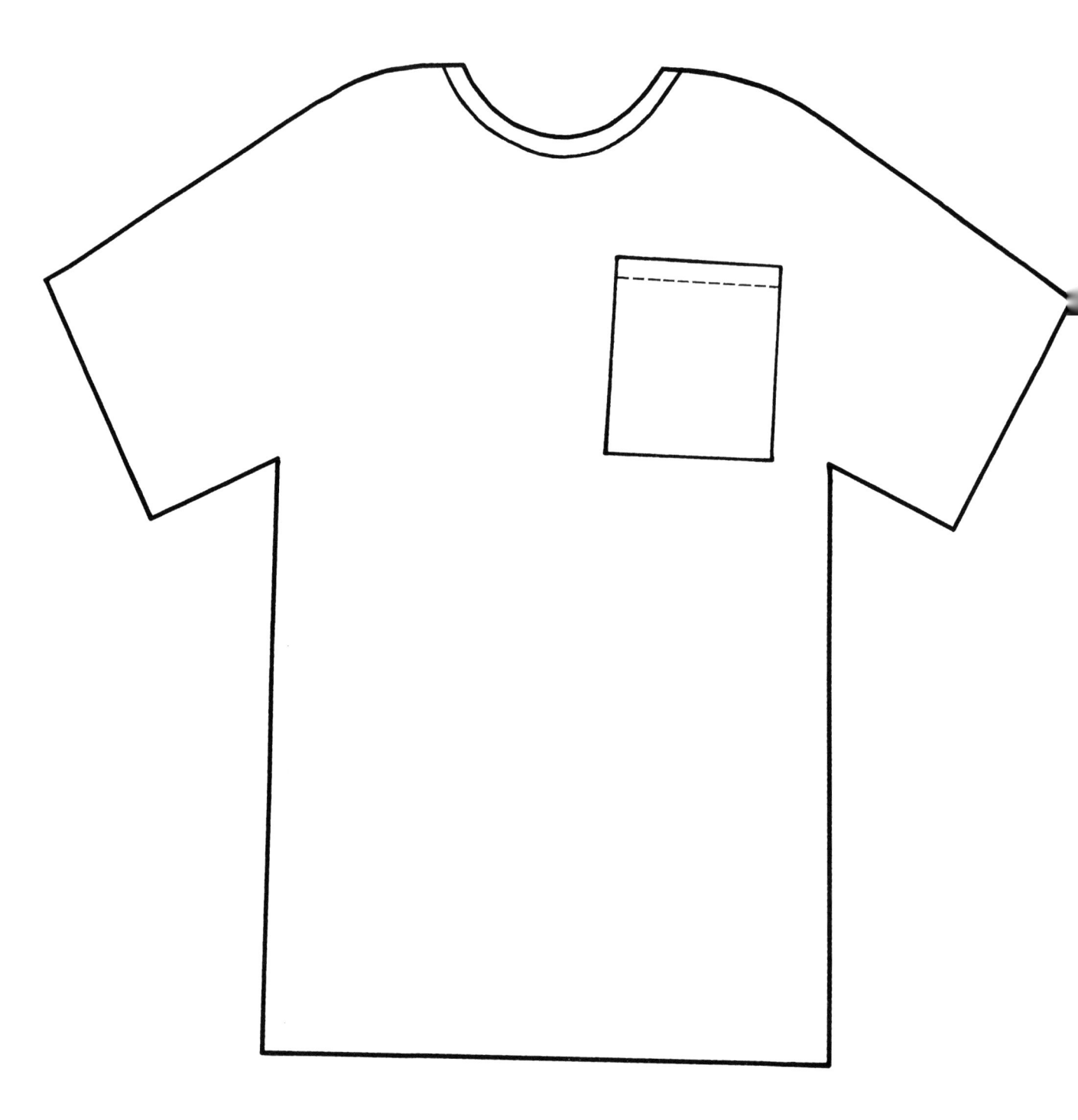

Reproducible. Copyright © 1999 Imaginart International, Inc.

Note

The next group of activities are modified from Level 3 to address Level 4 skills. You may want to refer to the Level 3 activities with the same names. Make sure that you and the child have played the Level 3 versions of these games before trying the modified version.

Follow the Path
Modified for Level 4

Purpose

To differentiate directional concepts on others. To give directional instructions to others.

Materials

Any reproducible *Follow the Path* grid map found on pages 62-69 and a wide-point highlighting marker

Procedure

- Choose a *Follow the Path* grid map to photocopy. There are eight themes to choose from: Mouse to Cheese, Rocket to Moon, Bee to Flower, Dog to Doghouse, Fish to Fishbowl, Frog to Lilly Pad, Bird to Nest, and Child to Bed. In the instructions below, the Rocket to the Moon theme is used as an example.

- Before the game, use the highlighting marker to draw a path from the start to the finish. Make sure to draw only horizontal and vertical lines. Use the grid lines as guides. Now you are ready to start the game.

- Sit across from the child so that you are facing each other. Orient the *Follow the Path* map so that you can see it; the child will perceive it as upside down.

- Tell the child, "I made a path from the rocket to the moon. I will place my finger on the rocket. Give me left, right, up and down instructions to get to the rocket. Remember to give the instructions from my point of view."

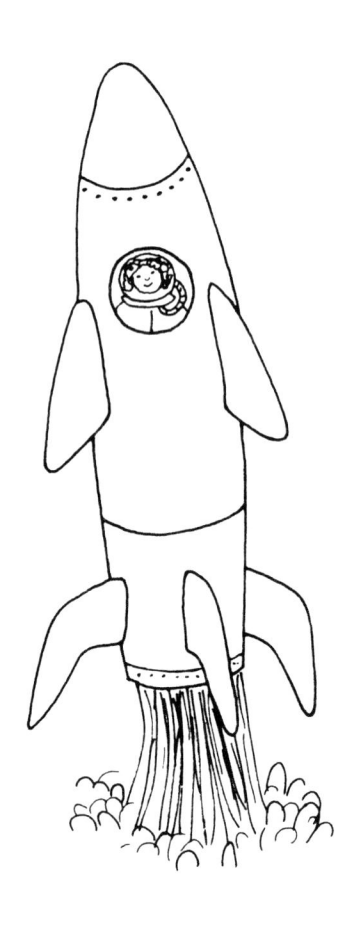

LEVEL 4—OTHERS AS A REFERENCE POINT

Observe

Is the child able to differentiate directional concepts on a person facing in the opposite direction? Can he give accurate directional instructions to a person facing in the opposite direction?

More Ideas

Allow the child to use the highlighting marker to draw the path.

Make a Map
Modified for Level 4

Purpose

To differentiate directional concepts on others. To give directional instructions to others.

Materials

Any reproducible *Make a Map* grid map found on pages 72-75, pencil and a sheet of lined paper

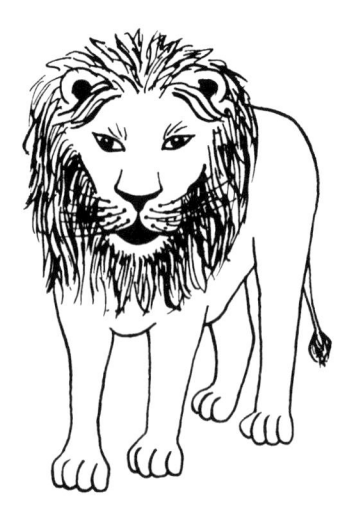

Procedure

- Choose a *Make a Map* grid map to photocopy. There are four themes to choose from: a Carnival, a Grocery Store, a Mall and a Zoo. In the instructions below, the Zoo theme is used as an example.

- Before the game, discuss the Zoo grid sheet with the child. Say, "Look at all of the places at the zoo that you can go to. Decide where you want to go. Use your pencil and paper to write the names of the places you want to go in the order you want to go to them. Here is an example:

    1) Snakes

    2) Lions

    3) Pandas"

- Sit across from the child so that you are facing each other. Orient the *Make a Map* grid map so that you can see it; the child will perceive it as upside down.

- Tell the child, "Let's see if you can send me to all of the places on your list. I will put my pencil on the starting square. Give me left, right, up and down instructions to go to each place in correct order. Remember to give the instructions from my point of view."

LEVEL 4—OTHERS AS A REFERENCE POINT

Observe

Is the child able to differentiate directional concepts on a person facing in the opposite direction? Can she give accurate directional instructions to a person facing in the opposite direction?

More Ideas

See if the child can direct you back to the starting square correctly.

Park Your Penny
Modified for Level 4

Purpose

To differentiate directional concepts on others. To give directional instructions to others.

Materials

Map of *Coinville, U.S.A.*, found on page 78, and 1 penny

Procedure

- Before the game, discuss the *Coinville, U.S.A.*, map with the child. Say, "This is a map of a town. Look at the streets, buildings and parking lots. Let's pretend that in Coinville people drive pennies instead of cars."

- Sit across from the child so that you are facing each other. Orient the *Coinville, U.S.A.* map so that you can see it; the child will perceive it as upside down.

- Tell the child, "Choose a location in Coinville and send me there. I will put my penny in the starting square. Give me left, right, up and down instructions to drive my penny to the location you chose. Remember to give the instructions from my point of view."

Observe

Is the child able to differentiate directional concepts on a person facing in the opposite direction? Can she give accurate directional instructions to a person facing in the opposite direction?

More Ideas

See if the child can direct you back to the starting square correctly.

Three-Ways Maze
Modified for Level 4

Purpose

To differentiate directional concepts on others.
To give directional instructions to others.

Materials

Reproducible *Three-Ways Maze* grid sheet found on page 96; and pink, blue and yellow highlighting markers

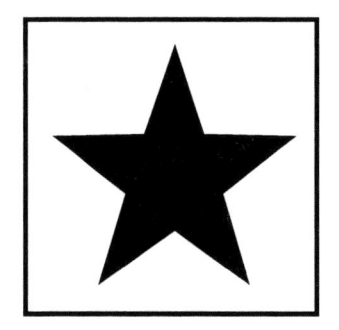

Procedure

- Photocopy the *Three-Ways Maze* grid sheet.

- Sit across from the child so that you are facing each other. Orient the *Three-Ways Maze* so that you can see it; the child will perceive it as upside down.

- Tell the child, "This maze has many different paths. All the paths lead to the star. Your job is to give me instructions to get to the star. You must find three different ways to send me to the star."

- Continue instructing the child by saying, "I will use the pink marker to make the first path. I will put the marker on Start #1. You give me left, right, up or down instructions to get to the star. Remember to give the instructions from my point of view."

- When you reach the star, say, "Now I will use the blue marker to trace a new path. I will begin the blue path at Start #2. You give me left, right, up or down instructions to get to the star. Try to avoid all of the pink paths. Remember to give the instructions from my point of view."

- When you reach the star, continue by saying, "Next, I will use the yellow marker to trace one more new path. I will begin the yellow path at Start #3. You give me left, right, up or down instructions to get to the star. This time try to avoid both the pink and blue paths while sending me to the star. Can you find a new path for me to take? Remember to give the instructions from my point of view."

LEVEL 4—OTHERS AS A REFERENCE POINT

Observe

Is the child able to differentiate directional concepts on a person facing in the opposite direction? Can she give accurate directional instructions to a person facing in the opposite direction?

More Ideas

See if the child can direct you back to the starting squares.

Fixed Reference Points:

Developing Readiness for Understanding North, East, South and West

Until now, *A Sense of Direction* has focused on understanding directional concepts relative to the self, objects and settings in the environment and from the perspective of others. Another stage in the development of direction sense occurs when spatial judgments are understood relative to fixed reference points.

Fixed reference points are the four cardinal directions: north, east, south and west. These fixed reference points never change. They remain constant no matter what position or location we are in. Understanding north, east, south and west is an advanced skill that many people find challenging even into adulthood. This skill is a necessary component of navigation, orienteering and wayfinding–or simply put, finding one's way in the world. Common examples of fixed reference point tasks include reading a map, driving to a new location or explaining directions to your house.

Although these skills are typically needed in adulthood, children can develop readiness skills for understanding fixed reference points that will help them in later years. A common misconception is that a child must simply learn how to read a compass in order to understand north, east, south and west. In her book, *The Sierra Club Wayfinding Book*, cultural geographer and cartographer Vicki McVey describes many other ways to teach children how to find their way in the world.

McVey explains that "Becoming a skilled wayfinder means learning how to pay attention to and make use of all your senses" (1989, p. 18). Long before the advent of the compass, people relied on smell, touch and hearing to provide clues to direction and location. Clues in nature also helped people find their way. Among these were the wind, stars, sun, moon and planets as well as landmarks in the environment.

Refining these observational skills by actively exploring the outside environment is the first step in understanding fixed reference points. Through exploration, the child learns to form cognitive maps of the environment. The cognitive map includes visual images of landmarks associated with specific locations. This information can be transferred onto paper as a map. By relating landmarks in the environment to locations on a map, the child can practice wayfinding. Through experience and repetition, the child can then learn to describe the location of landmarks in the environment relative to the cardinal directions on the map.

Using a map requires practice like any other skill. Here are some strategies that beginners can use to develop map skills:

- Learn to turn the map so that north on the map is actually pointing north in the environment.

- Look for natural landmarks. Find them on the map and mark their location. Mark your position relative to the landmarks.

- When walking, take a "back bearing" by looking back at the place you just left.

- When you are in a city, first study a map to see how streets are laid out. Streets are usually oriented north and south and east and west.

- Try to notice city landmarks. Keep track of your position relative to landmarks at all times.

Many activities in *A Sense of Direction* can be modified to practice wayfinding and map skills. *Looking for Landmarks* (page 140) is an excellent activity to teach children how to become more aware of their environment. It also promotes wayfinding skills as children learn to associate landmarks with routes and changes in direction. The two-dimensional grid games can also be modified to teach concepts of north, east, south and west. Simply add the cardinal directions to the grid sheets. Instead of saying "left, right, up or down," the child can practice giving and following "north, east, south and west" instructions. The following activities can be modified in this way:

Follow the Path	Page 60
Make a Map	Page 70
Park Your Penny	Page 76
Three-Ways Maze	Page 94

Games, Sports and Compensatory Strategies to Build Directional Skills

To be truly effective, the development of functional directional skills must extend beyond the therapy setting. Children with directional confusion must be taught "survival strategies" to help them understand and use directional concepts. Although children with sensorimotor delays or processing deficits benefit greatly from remedial techniques, teaching problem-solving and compensatory strategies should represent a major component of treatment.

The activities in *A Sense of Direction* incorporate remedial, problem solving and compensatory techniques. There are, however, many other activities available to children that support the development of directional skills. Among these are games and sports.

Games

The following is a listing of commercially available games that support the development of directional skills and spatial concepts:

- Twister
- Big Hands and Feet
- TrickyFingers
- Battleship
- Etch-a-Sketch
- The A-Mazing Labyrinth
- Memory

Other traditional games that promote the ability to follow directions include
- Simon Says
- Mother May I
- Hokey Pokey

Computer games with CD ROM capacity allow the child to explore virtual environments or change the positions of objects in space. Others build map-reading skills. Some excellent computer games for children that promote spatial concepts and directional skills are

Lego Island by Mindscape, Inc., 88 Rowland Way, Novato, CA 94945

The Lost Mind of Dr. Brain by Sierra On-Line, Inc., 3380 146th Place SE, Suite 300, Bellevue, WA 98007

Make a Map by Panasonic Interactive Media, 4701 Patrick Henry Drive, Suite 1101, Santa Clara, CA 95054

Where in the World is Carmen Sandiego? by Broderbund Software, Inc., P.O. Box 6125, Novato, CA 94948

Where in the U.S.A. is Carmen Sandiego? by Broderbund Software, Inc., P.O. Box 6125, Novato, CA 94948

Trails Adventure Set by The Learning Company, Inc., TLC Headquarters, One Athenaeum St., Cambridge, MA 02142

Sports

Active participation in sports can improve directional skills. Children experiencing directional confusion often avoid sports because of uncertainty and embarrassment. Team sports can be particularly difficult for these children. Sports that allow children to learn at their own pace, on the other hand, are good choices for those with directional confusion. A patient and understanding instructor can instill both skill and confidence, helping children overcome their uncertainties. The following is a list of some sports that support the development of directional skills:

- martial arts
- gymnastics
- hiking
- rock climbing
- sailing
- swimming
- biking
- skating
- skiing
- yoga

Orienteering is a sport dedicated entirely to the development of directional skills. Orienteering is the sport of cross-country navigation using a map and a compass. The sport of orienteering originated in Scandinavia in 1919 where scout leader, Ernst Killander, first developed a cross-country treasure hunt incorporating skills of land navigation and fitness training. Orienteering came to the United States in the late 1960s. The sport has grown steadily since the 1970s when the first United States Orienteering Championships were held at Southern Illinois University.

Orienteering groups set up special courses in parks. They provide a detailed topographical orienteering map of the course including landmarks such as boulders and streams. They even set up special beginners' courses and provide orienteering instruction for beginners and children. Even young children can follow a string course while looking at a picture map (Nash, 1995).

General information about orienteering and a list of orienteering clubs throughout the country can be obtained by sending a self-addressed, stamped envelope to

The United States Orienteering Federation

P.O. Box 1444

Forest Park, GA 30298

(404) 363-2110

Web site: www.us.orienteering.org/

Compensatory Strategies

Compensatory and problem-solving strategies help children with directional confusion overcome their weaknesses. Rather than feeling overwhelmed and discouraged, these "survival skills" empower children to organize spatial information for functional use. Examples of a few compensatory and problem-solving strategies are listed below (Levine, 1991 and McVay, 1998).

- Wear jewelry or a watch on the left hand to differentiate left from right.

- Use the left index finger and thumb to form an "L" to differentiate left from right.

- If right-handed, remember the phrase "I write with my right."

- Provide footprints and handprints marked "L" and "R" for children to put their hands and feet on.

- During left and right games, place a red sticker on the right hand and foot. Teach children to remember the phrase "Red is for right."

- Pair directional arrows with directional words such as, "up, down, left and right."

- When walking in a new place, notice landmarks. Practice visualizing the landmarks to remember them the next time.

- Become aware of sensory clues when you are exploring a new place. Notice the wind, the angle of the sun, noises and scents. Remember that the sun rises in the east and sets in the west.

- When going to a new location, preview a map of the area. Draw your route on the map with a highlighting marker. Circle landmarks to look for along your route.

- When using a map, hold it so that north on the map actually points to north in the environment.

- When traveling in an unfamiliar city, always carry your home address and phone number as well as the address and phone number of your destination.

Appendix

Instructions for Quick Screen and Pre-/Post-Tests

Quick Screen

The *Sense of Direction* Quick Screen (page 190) is an easy way to determine a child's directional skills. It is a brief checklist of 10 items sequenced by level of difficulty. Next to each item is an approximate age range for skill acquisition. It is important to note that the age ranges listed are not based on empirical data and therefore should not be used as a standardized measure of development. Rather, the Quick Screen is a tool designed to approximate a current level of function, to determine the need for intervention and to guide treatment planning.

To administer the Quick Screen, begin with Item 1 and continue until you have reached the item corresponding to the child's chronological age range. Make sure to orient yourself as noted in the instructions. You will need the Star Path (page 195) for items 7, 8 and 10. After giving each instruction, count-off 3 seconds by silently saying "one-one thousand, two-one thousand, three-one thousand." This technique, described in the *Southern California Sensory Integration Right and Left Discrimination Test* (Ayres, 1979), allows the practitioner to estimate response time. A response time within 3 seconds suggests that the skill is well integrated on an automatic level; a delayed response time of more than 3 seconds suggests that the child is over reliant on cognition or compensatory clues. Use the spaces provided to mark each correct response with a "+" and each incorrect response with a "-." Circle every "+" or "-" response that exceeds 3 seconds. Use the results of the screening in conjunction with clinical observations to determine if the child's directional skill development: 1) appears to be within normal limits for his age level, 2) appears to be below age level or 3) is delayed in response time.

Pre-/Post-Tests

The *Sense of Direction* Pre-/Post-Tests are tools to measure progress. There are four pre-/post-tests, each corresponding to a level of directional skill development described in *A Sense of Direction*. They may be used by practitioners to determine if a child is ready to try more challenging activities at the next level. Or, they may be used to document skill acquisition for the purposes of reevaluation and treatment planning.

Unlike the Quick Screen, each pre-/post-test item is given a numerical point value. The pre-test score is then compared with the post-test score to measure progress. Like the Quick Screen, "+" or "-" responses that are delayed for more than 3 seconds are circled. The total number of delayed responses at the time of the pre-test is then compared to the total number at the time of post-test. This will help the practitioner determine if skills are integrated on an automatic level. Skills at each level should be automatic before proceeding to the next level.

When administering test items, make sure that you are oriented as noted in the instructions. The pre-/post-tests for Level 1 and Level 2 do not require materials. You will need the following materials for the Level 3 and Level 4 pre-/post-tests:

    Level 3 - Star Grid, page 196, small wooden block and a Wall Star,
        page 197
    Level 4 - Star Path, page 195

A Sense of Direction–Quick Screen

Name: _____ Teacher/Grade: _____

Date of Screening: _____ Date of Birth: _____ Chronological Age: ____

Referral Information: _____
_____
_____

MATERIALS: Pencil; a Star Path for items 7, 8 and 10.

INSTRUCTIONS: Stand facing the child for items 1 - 6. Sit at a table across from the child for items 7 - 10. Indicate a correct response with a **+**. Indicate an incorrect response with a **-**. If the child takes longer than 3 seconds to respond, circle the + or - score. **Age ranges for screening items are approximations** to be considered along with referral information and response time in determining need for further testing.

_____ 1. Touch the **top** of your head. Touch the **bottom** of your foot. (ages 3 - 6)
(Both responses must be correct for + score.)

_____ 2. Touch the **front** of your body. Touch the **back** of your body. (ages 3 - 6)
(Both responses must be correct for + score.)

_____ 3. Walk **forward**. Walk **backward**. (ages 3 - 6)
(Both responses must be correct for + score.)

_____ 4. Show me your **left** hand. (ages 6 - 7)

_____ 5. Touch your **right** ear. (ages 6 - 7)

_____ 6. With your **right** hand, touch your **left** knee. (ages 7 - 8)

_____ 7. Write your name in the **top left-hand** corner of the paper. (ages 8 - 10)

_____ 8. Place your finger on the dot and follow the path to the star. Tell me which way you are going to follow the path: right, left, up or down. (ages 8 - 10)

_____ 9. Now look at me and point to **my left** hand. (ages 9 - 11)

Turn the Star Path so that it is oriented correctly for you.

_____ 10. This time I will put my finger on the dot. You tell me which way to go to reach the star: right, left, up or down. (ages 9 - 12)

Appears within normal limits for age level _____

Appears below age level _____

Response time exceeds 3 seconds, suggesting delay _____

Reproducible. Copyright © 1999 Imaginart International, Inc.

A Sense of Direction – Pre-/Post-Test

Level 1 - Body Awareness
The ability to differentiate and locate body parts in response to verbal request.

Name:_____ Teacher/Grade:_____

MATERIALS: None
INSTRUCTIONS: Indicate correct responses with a +. Indicate incorrect responses with a -. If the child takes longer than 3 seconds to respond, circle the + or -.

Items	Pre-Test Date _____	Post-Test Date _____
1. Touch your eyes.	_____	_____
2. Touch your mouth.	_____	_____
3. Touch your ears.	_____	_____
4. Touch your nose.	_____	_____
5. Touch your hands.	_____	_____
6. Touch your feet.	_____	_____
7. Touch your stomach.	_____	_____
8. Touch your back.	_____	_____
9. Touch your arm.	_____	_____
10. Touch your leg.	_____	_____
11. Touch your head.	_____	_____
12. Touch your knees.	_____	_____
13. Touch your elbow.	_____	_____
14. Touch your shoulder.	_____	_____
15. Touch your waist.	_____	_____
16. Touch your hips.	_____	_____
17. Touch your wrist.	_____	_____
18. Touch your ankle.	_____	_____
19. Touch your neck.	_____	_____
20. Touch your chest.	_____	_____

Score 5 points for each + response
Score 0 points for each - response
Maximum score = 100 points   Pre-Test Score   Post-Test Score

Total Score: _____   _____

Total number of circled delayed responses: _____   _____

Reproducible. Copyright © 1999 Imaginart International, Inc.

A Sense of Direction – Pre-/Post-Test

Level 2 - Self as a Reference Point
The ability to differentiate left/right, top/bottom and front/back on self. The ability to follow left/right, up/down and forward/backward instructions relative to self.

Name:_____ Teacher/Grade:_____

MATERIALS: None

INSTRUCTIONS: *Indicate correct responses with a +. Indicate incorrect responses with a -. If the child takes longer than 3 seconds to respond, circle the + or -.*

Items	Pre-Test Date	Post-Test Date
1. Reach up.	_____	_____
2. Reach down.	_____	_____
3. Touch the top of your head.	_____	_____
4. Touch the bottom of your foot.	_____	_____
5. Touch your right ear.	_____	_____
6. Touch your left eye.	_____	_____
7. Touch your left knee.	_____	_____
8. Touch your right foot.	_____	_____
9. Touch the back of your body.	_____	_____
10. Touch the front of your body.	_____	_____
11. Walk backward.	_____	_____
12. Walk to your right.	_____	_____
13. Walk forward.	_____	_____
14. Walk to your left.	_____	_____
15. With your right hand, touch your right knee.	_____	_____
16. With your right hand, touch your left shoulder.	_____	_____
17. With your left hand, touch your left foot.	_____	_____
18. With your left hand, touch right elbow.	_____	_____
19. Walk forward two steps, then walk right two steps.	_____	_____
20. Walk backward two steps, then walk left two steps.	_____	_____

Score 5 points for each + response
Score 0 points for each - response
Maximum score = 100 points

	Pre-Test Score	Post-Test Score
Total Score:	_____	_____
Total number of circled delayed responses:	_____	_____

Reproducible. Copyright © 1999 Imaginart International, Inc.

A Sense of Direction – Pre-/Post-Test

Level 3 - Environment as a Reference Point
The ability to differentiate directional concepts and follow directional instructions in both two- and three-dimensional space.

Name: _____ Teacher/Grade: _____

MATERIALS: *Star Grid for items 1 - 10, a small wooden cube for items 11 - 16 and a Wall Star for items 17 - 20.*
INSTRUCTIONS: *Indicate correct responses with a +. Indicate incorrect responses with a -. If the child takes longer than 3 seconds to respond, circle the + or -.*

Items	Pre-Test Date	Post-Test Date
	_____	_____

Give the child a copy of the Star Grid.
1. Point to any star at the top of the paper.
2. Point to any star at the bottom of the paper.
3. Point to the star in the top right corner.
4. Point to the star in the bottom left corner.
5. Point to the star in the top left corner.
6. Point to the star in the bottom right corner.

Touch the star in the center and tell the child, "Put your finger on this star."

7. Slide your finger up one square.
8. Slide your finger left one square.
9. Slide your finger down one square.
10. Slide your finger right one square.

Place the small wooden cube on the table in front of the child.

11. Touch the top of the cube.
12. Touch the right side of the cube.
13. Touch the front of the cube.
14. Touch the bottom of the cube.
15. Touch the left side of the cube.
16. Touch the back of the cube.

Tape the Wall Star at the front of the room and tell the child, "Face the star."

17. Walk to the front of the room.
18. Walk to the left of the room.
19. Walk to the back of the room.
20. Walk to the right of the room.

Score 5 points for each + response
Score 0 points for each - response
Maximum score = 100 points   Pre-Test Score   Post-Test Score

Total Score:
Total number of circled delayed responses:

Reproducible. Copyright © 1999 Imaginart International, Inc.

A Sense of Direction – Pre-/Post-Test

Level 4 - Others as a Reference Point
The ability to differentiate directional concepts on others and to give directional instructions to others.

Name: _____ Teacher/Grade: _____

MATERIALS: Star Path for items 11 - 15.

INSTRUCTIONS: Stand next to the child for items 1 and 2. Stand facing the child for items 3 - 10. Sit at a table across from the child and position the Star Path so that it is oriented correctly for you during items 11 - 15. Indicate correct responses with a +. Indicate incorrect responses with a -. If the child takes longer than 3 seconds to respond, circle the + or -.

Items	Pre-Test Date	Post-Test Date

Stand next to the child.
1. Point to my left arm.
2. Point to my right arm.
   Proceed with test only if items 1 and 2 are +.
   Stand facing the child.
3. Point to my right arm.
4. Point to my left arm.
5. Point to the front of my body.
6. Point to the back of my body.
7. *Walk forward.* Say, "Am I walking forward or backward?"
8. *Walk backward.* Say, "Am I walking forward or backward?"
9. *Sidestep left.* Say, "Am I walking right or left?"
10. *Sidestep right.* Say, "Am I walking right or left?"
    Sit across from the child. Referring to the Star Path, say, "I will put the paper in front of me and place my finger on the dot. You tell me which way to go to reach the star: right, left, up or down."
11. Correct response: up
12. Correct response: right
13. Correct response: up
14. Correct response: left
15. Correct response: down
16. **BONUS ITEM WORTH 25 POINTS:** Consider your setting and choose a location in another part of the building such as an office, gymnasium or library. Tell the child, "Pretend that I don't know where the library is. Give me instructions to get there. Remember to use landmarks and direction words such as left and right in your instructions."

Score 5 points for each + response
Score 0 points for each - response
Maximum score = 100 points (75 points + bonus)

Pre-Test Score   Post-Test Score

Total Score:

Total number of circled delayed responses:

Reproducible. Copyright © 1999 Imaginart International, Inc.

Star Path

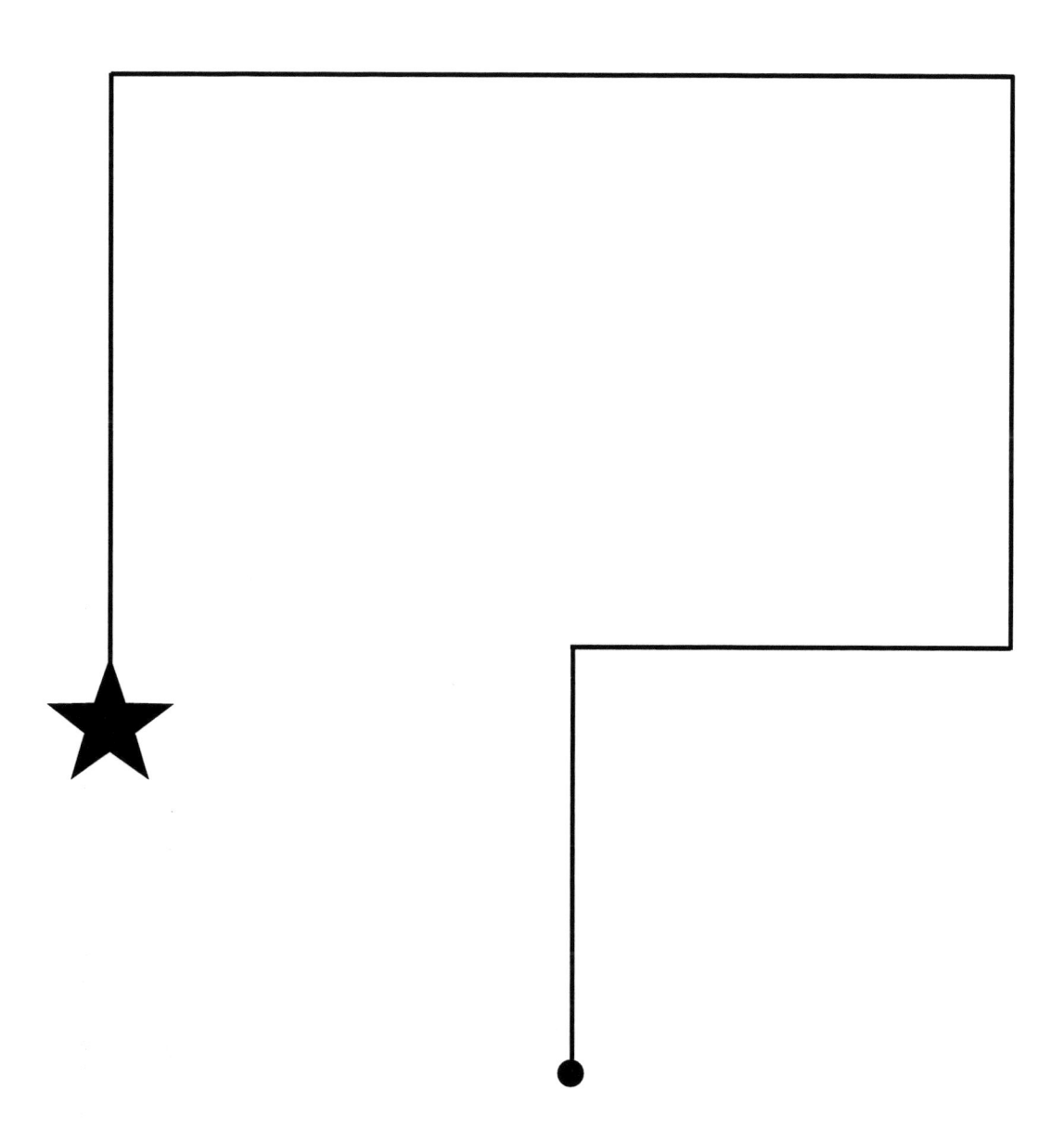

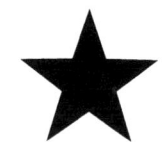

Star Grid

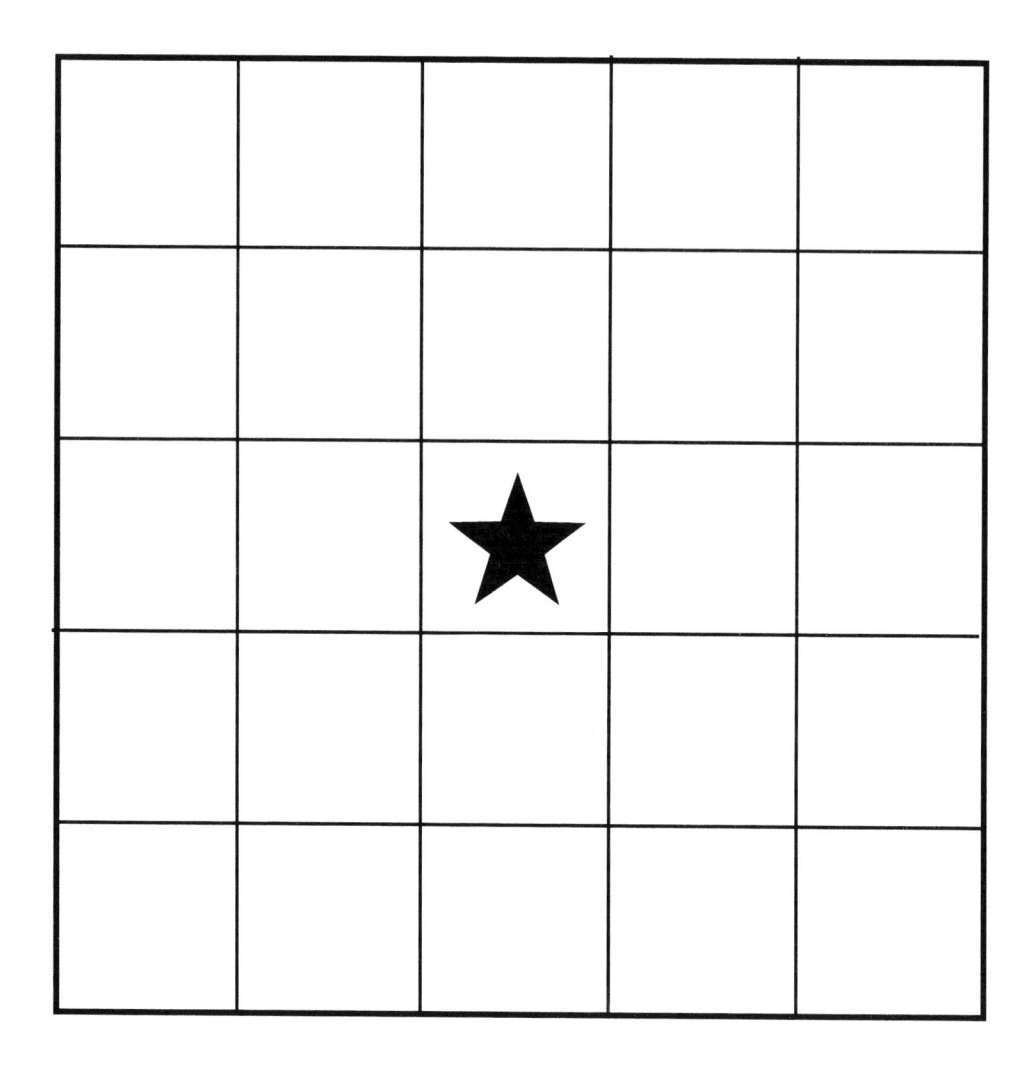

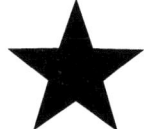

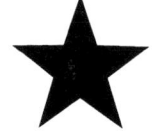

Wall Star

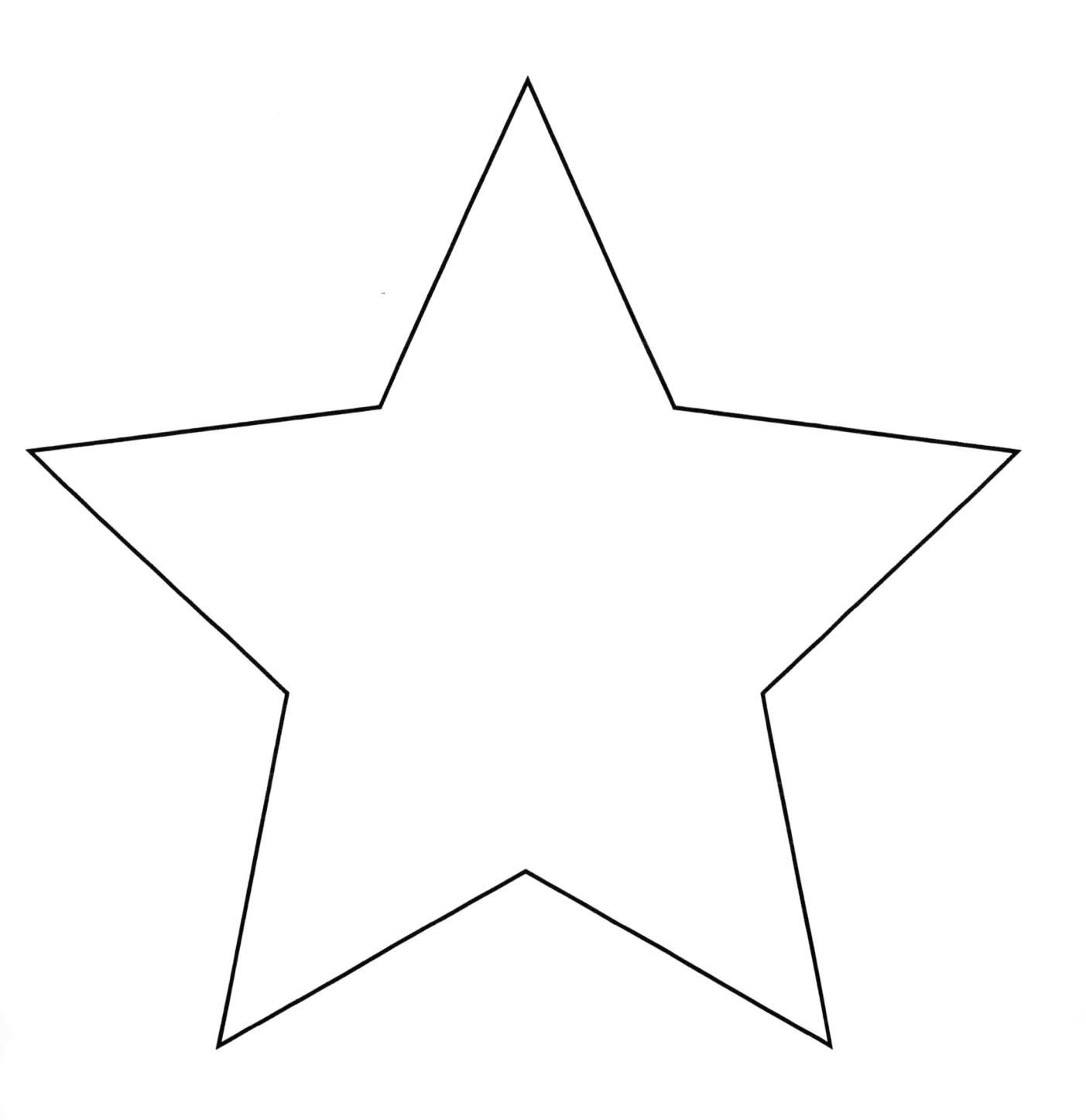

Reproducible. Copyright © 1999 Imaginart International, Inc.

197

A Sense of Direction – Goals and Objectives

Sample Goals

Goal: To improve functional directional skills for greater independence in the school environment.

Goal: To improve functional directional skills for greater independence in the community environment.

Goal: To improve functional directional skills for greater independence in activities of daily living.

Sample Objectives

Level 1 Objective

Who - Name
What - will demonstrate body awareness
How - by differentiating and locating body parts in response to verbal request
Where - during the selected activities in the _____ setting
When - in _____ out of _____ trials

Level 2 Objective

Who - Name
What - will demonstrate understanding of directional concepts relative to self
How - by differentiating (right/left, up/down, front/back) on self and following (right/left, up/down, forward/backward) instructions relative to self
Where - during the selected activities in the _____ setting
When - in _____ out of _____ trials

Level 3 Objective

Who - Name
What - will demonstrate understanding of directional concepts relative to the environment
How - by differentiating (right/left, top/bottom, front/back) and following (right/left, up/down, forward/backward) instructions in two- and three-dimensional space
Where - during the selected activities in the _____ setting
When - in _____ out of _____ trials

Level 4 Objective

Who - Name
What - will demonstrate understanding of directional concepts relative to others
How - by differentiating (right/left, top/bottom, front/back) on others and giving (right/left, up/down, forward/backward) instructions to others
Where - during the selected activities in the _____ setting
When - in _____ out of _____ trials

Reproducible. Copyright © 1999 Imaginart International, Inc.

Combined Level Objective

Who - Name
What - will demonstrate understanding of directional concepts relative to self, environment and others
How - by differentiating between and following and giving directional instructions (right/left, up/down, top/bottom, front/back, forward/backward)
Where - during the selected activities in the _____ setting
When - in _____ out of _____ trials

Examples of Alternate Objectives

Who - Name
What - will demonstrate improved spatial organization skills
How - by following directional instructions (right/left, up/down, top/bottom, front/back, forward/backward)
Where - during the selected activities in the _____ setting
When - in _____ out of _____ trials

Who - Name
What - will direct others to a designated goal
How - by giving accurate right/left, forward/backward instructions
Where - during the selected activities in the _____ setting
When - in _____ out of _____ trials

Who - Name
What - will organize paperwork
How - by writing in the designated right/left, top/bottom, front/back area of the paper
Where - during the selected activities in the _____ setting
When - in _____ out of _____ trials

Reproducible. Copyright © 1999 Imaginart International, Inc.

A Sense of Direction – Individual Planning and Progress Guide

Name: _____ Date of Annual Review: _____

Goal: _____

Objective #1

What: _____

How: _____

Where: _____

When: _____

Objective #2

What: _____

How: _____

Where: _____

When: _____

Objective #3

What: _____

How: _____

Where: _____

When: _____

Objective #4

What: _____

How: _____

Where: _____

When: _____

Plan for First Quarter

Week	Obj. #	Level	Activity	Progress − ↑ +
1.				
2.				
3.				
4.				
5.				
6.				
7.				
8.				
9.				

Key: − (objective not met)   ↑ (progressing toward objective)   + (objective met)

Reproducible. Copyright © 1999 Imaginart International, Inc.

Plan for Second Quarter

Week	Obj. #	Level	Activity	Progress - ↑ +
1.				
2.				
3.				
4.				
5.				
6.				
7.				
8.				
9.				

Key: - (objective not met) ↑ (progressing toward objective) + (objective met)

Plan for Third Quarter

Week	Obj. #	Level	Activity	Progress - ↑ +
1.				
2.				
3.				
4.				
5.				
6.				
7.				
8.				
9.				

Key: - (objective not met) ↑ (progressing toward objective) + (objective met)

Plan for Fourth Quarter

Week	Obj. #	Level	Activity	Progress - ↑ +
1.				
2.				
3.				
4.				
5.				
6.				
7.				
8.				
9.				

Key: - (objective not met) ↑ (progressing toward objective) + (objective met)

Reproducible. Copyright © 1999 Imaginart International, Inc.

Sample Individual Planning and Progress Guide

Name: **Student**
Date of Annual Review: **00-00-00**
Goal: **To improve functional directional skills for independence in the school environment**

Objective #1
What: understand directional concepts relative to SELF
How: by differentiating & following R/L instructions
Where: during selected activities in therapy setting
When: in 10 out of 10 trials

Objective #2
What: understand directional concepts relative to ENVIRONMENT
How: by differentiating & following R/L instructions in 2-D & 3-D space
Where: during selected activities in inclusive setting
When: in 10 out of 10 trials

Objective #3
What: understand directional concepts relative to OTHERS
How: by differentiating & giving R/L instructions to others
Where: during selected activities in inclusive setting
When: in 7 out of 10 trials

Objective #4
What:
How:
Where:
When:

Plan for First Quarter

Week	Obj. #	Level	Activity	Progress (− ↑ +)
1. 9-1	1	2	Administer Level 2 Pre-Test	
2. 9-8	1	2	Crumple & Leaning Tower	−
3. 9-15	1	2	Make-Believe Hospital - 2	↑
4. 9-22	1	2	High 5's & Keep Your Eye on the Ball	↑
5. 9-29	1	2	High 5's & Where is the Sticker?	↑
6. 10-6	1	2	Mud Bath & Where is the Sticker?	↑
7. 10-13	1	2	High 5's & L/R Coin Sorting	+
8. 10-20	1	2	Keep Your Eye on the Ball & Tapping	+
9. 10-27	1	2	Administer Level 2 Post-Test	

Key: − (objective not met)   ↑ (progressing toward objective)   + (objective met)

Plan for Second Quarter

Week	Obj. #	Level	Activity	Progress − ↑ +
1. 11-3	2	3	Administer Level 3 Pre-Test	
2. 11-10	2	3	Follow the Path	↑
3. 11-17	2	3	Park Your Penny & Secret Door	↑
4. 11-24	2	3	3-Ways Maze	+
5. 12-1	2	3	File Cabinet	↑
6. 12-8	2	3	Prairie Dog Town	+
7. 12-15	2	3	Make a Map- Zoo & Mall	+
8. 1-5	2	3	Make a Map- Carnival & Store	+
9. 1-12	2	3	Floor Grid: Robots & Memory Match	↑

Plan for Third Quarter

Week	Obj. #	Level	Activity	Progress − ↑ +
1. 1-19	2	3	Floor Grid-Sticker Hunt	↑
2. 1-26	2	3	Animal Parade-grid maps and floor grid	+
3. 2-2	2	3	Mixed-Up Socks-grid maps and floor grid	+
4. 2-9	2	3	Mail Delivery-grid maps and floor grid	+
5. 2-16	2	3	Secret Word-grid maps and floor grid	↑
6. 2-23	2	3	Secret Word- repeat	+
7. 3-2	2	3	Plan for trip to museum	+
8. 3-9	2	3	Class trip-Looking for Landmarks	+
9. 3-23	2	3	Level 3 Post-Test	

Plan for Fourth Quarter

Week	Obj. #	Level	Activity	Progress − ↑ +
1. 3-30	3	4	Administer Level 4 Pre-Test	
2. 4-6	3	4	Picture Poses & Follow the Path-4	−
3. 4-13	3	4	Statue Maker & Park Your Penny-4	↑
4. 4-20	3	4	Paper People Cut-Outs	+
5. 4-27	3	4	3-Ways Maze-4 & Make a Map-4	+
6. 5-4	3	4	Design a Pocket T-shirt	+
7. 5-11	3	4	Plan for trip to zoo	+
8. 5-18	3	4	Class trip-Looking for Landmarks	+
9. 5-25	3	4	Level 4 Post-Test	

Key: − (objective not met)   ↑ (progressing toward objective)   + (objective met)

APPENDIX

Follow the Path

Make a Map

Start

16–Square Grid

Start			

Reproducible. Copyright © 1999 Imaginart International, Inc.

Three-Ways Maze

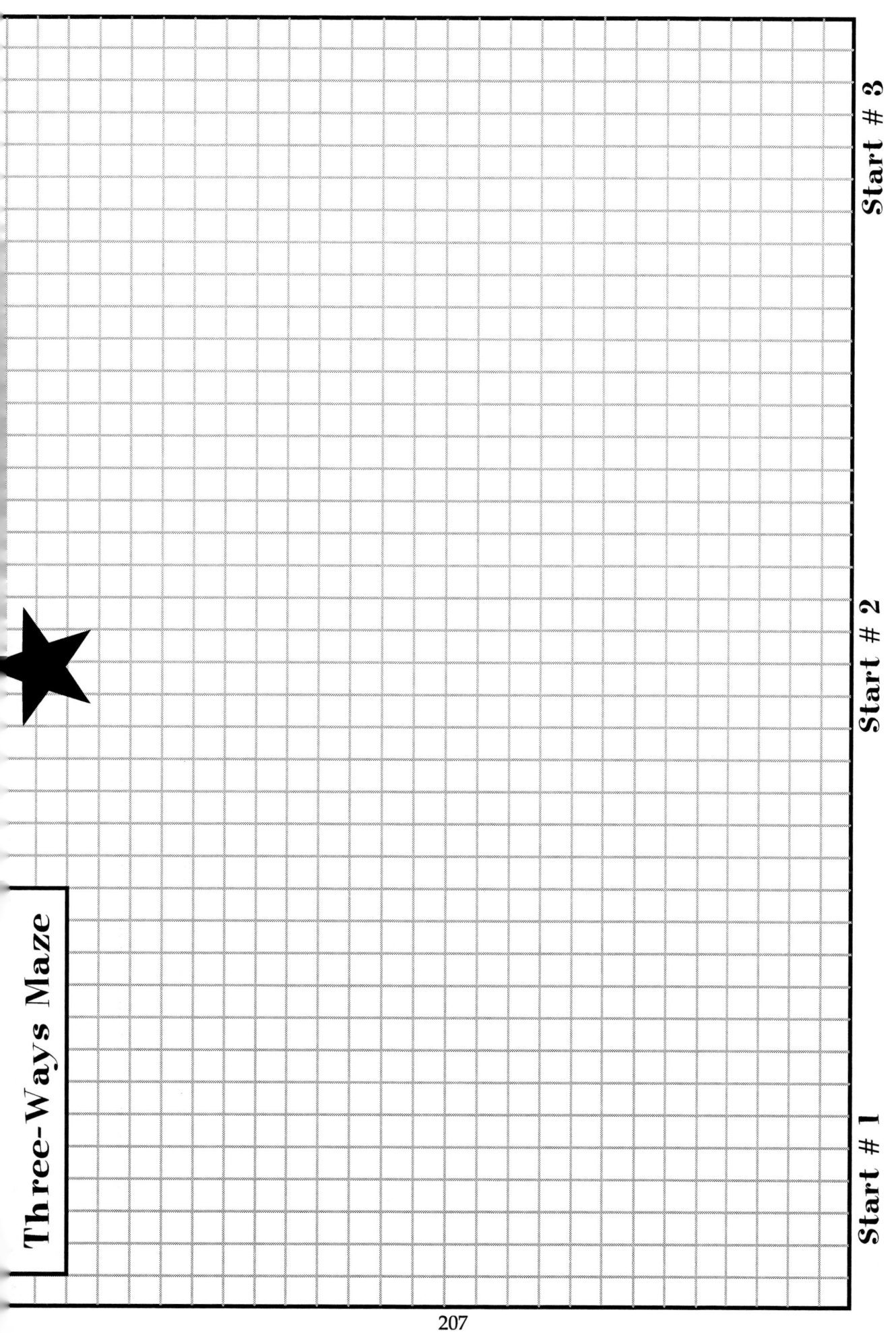

Start # 1   Start # 2   Start # 3

Secret Door

Start

Samples of Completed Grid Maps

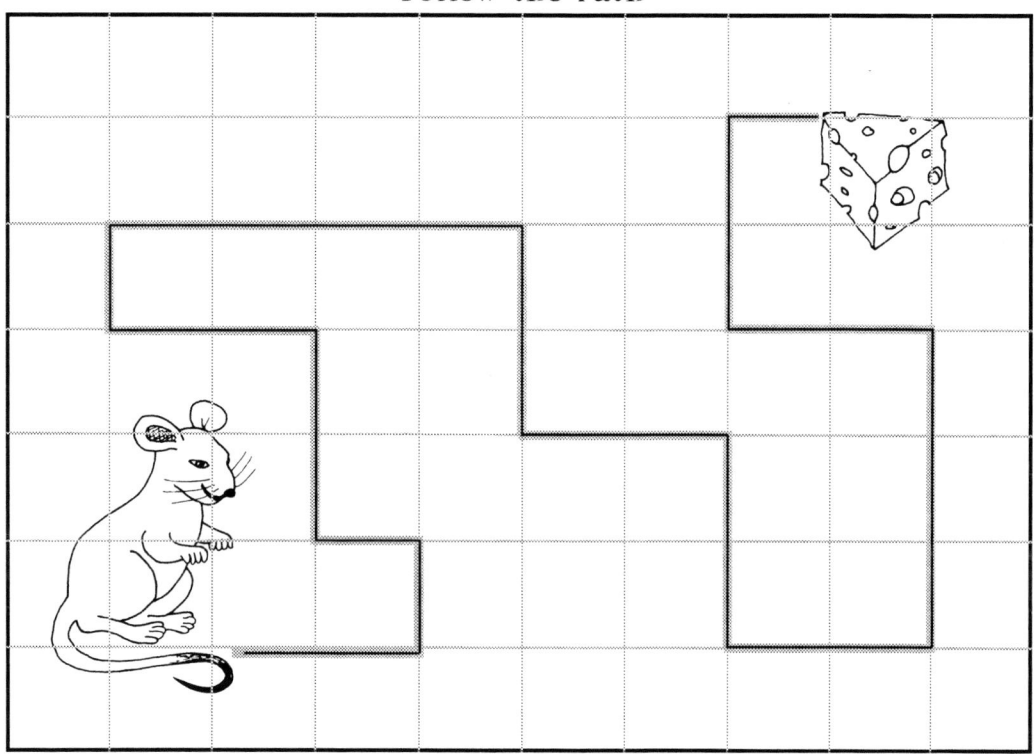

Follow the Path

Carnival

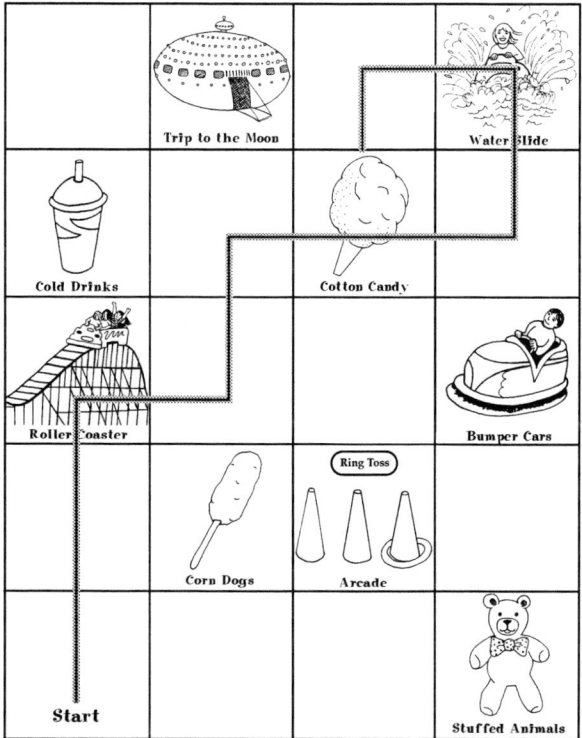

Make a Map

APPENDIX

209

Prairie Dog Town

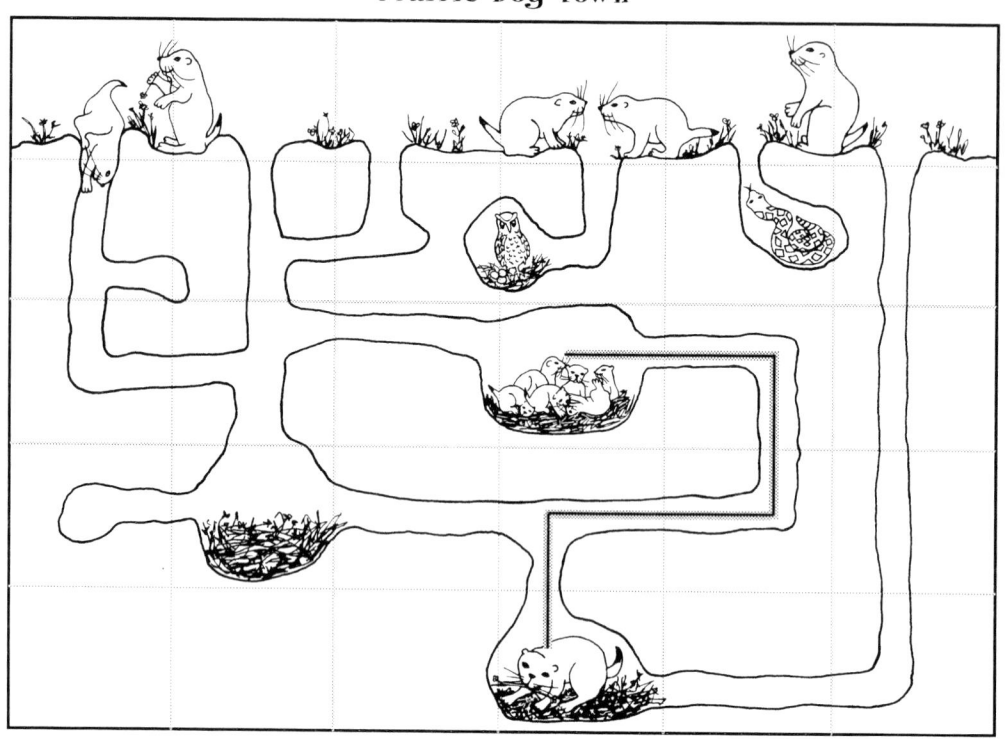

Animal Parade

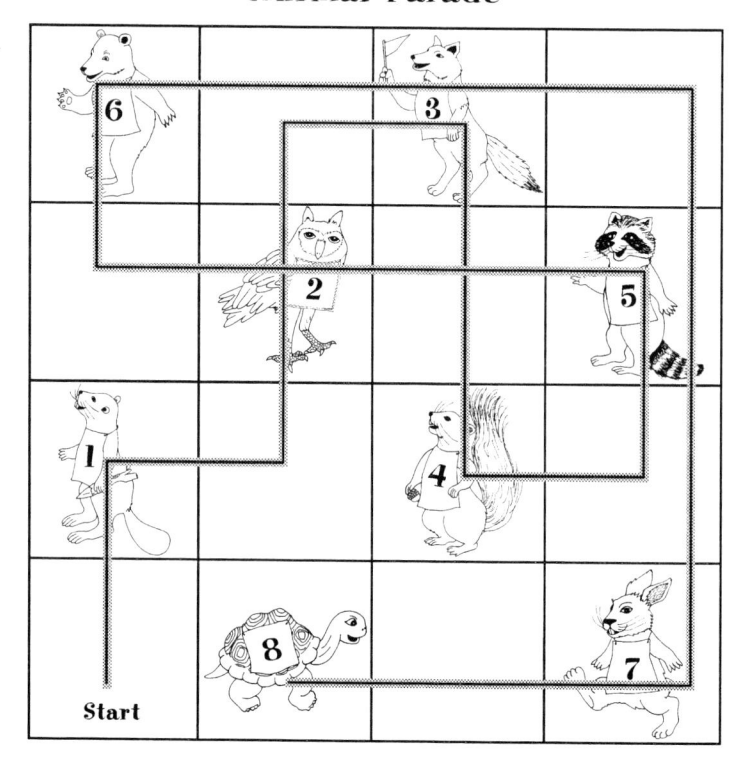

APPENDIX

Mixed-Up Socks

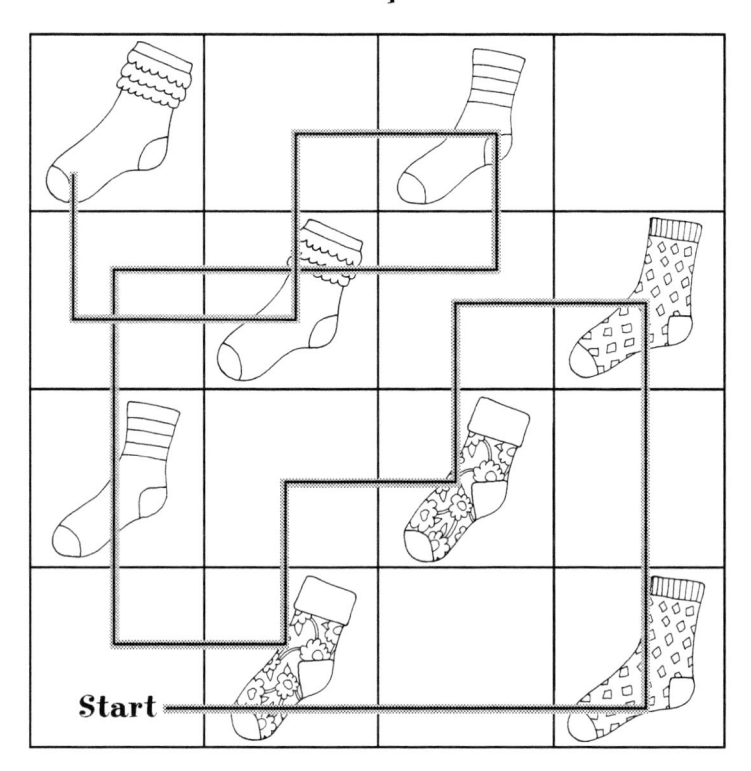

Secret Word

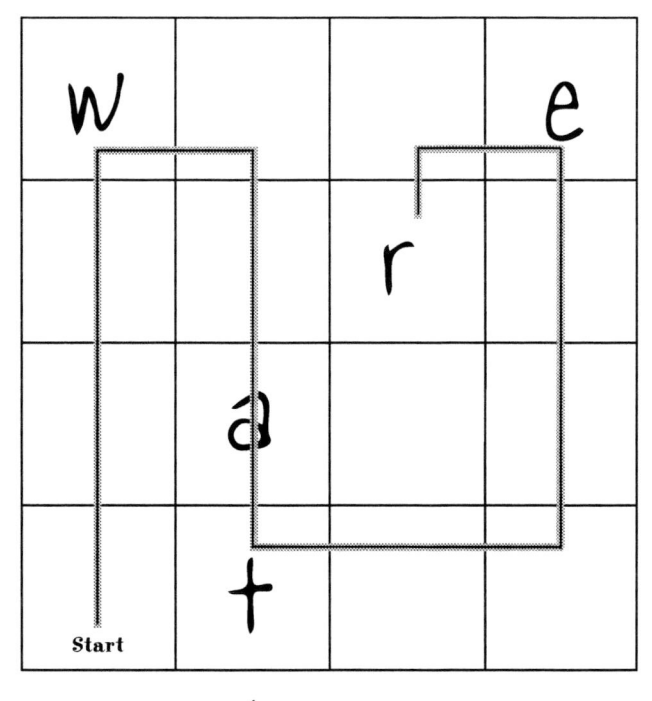

water

APPENDIX

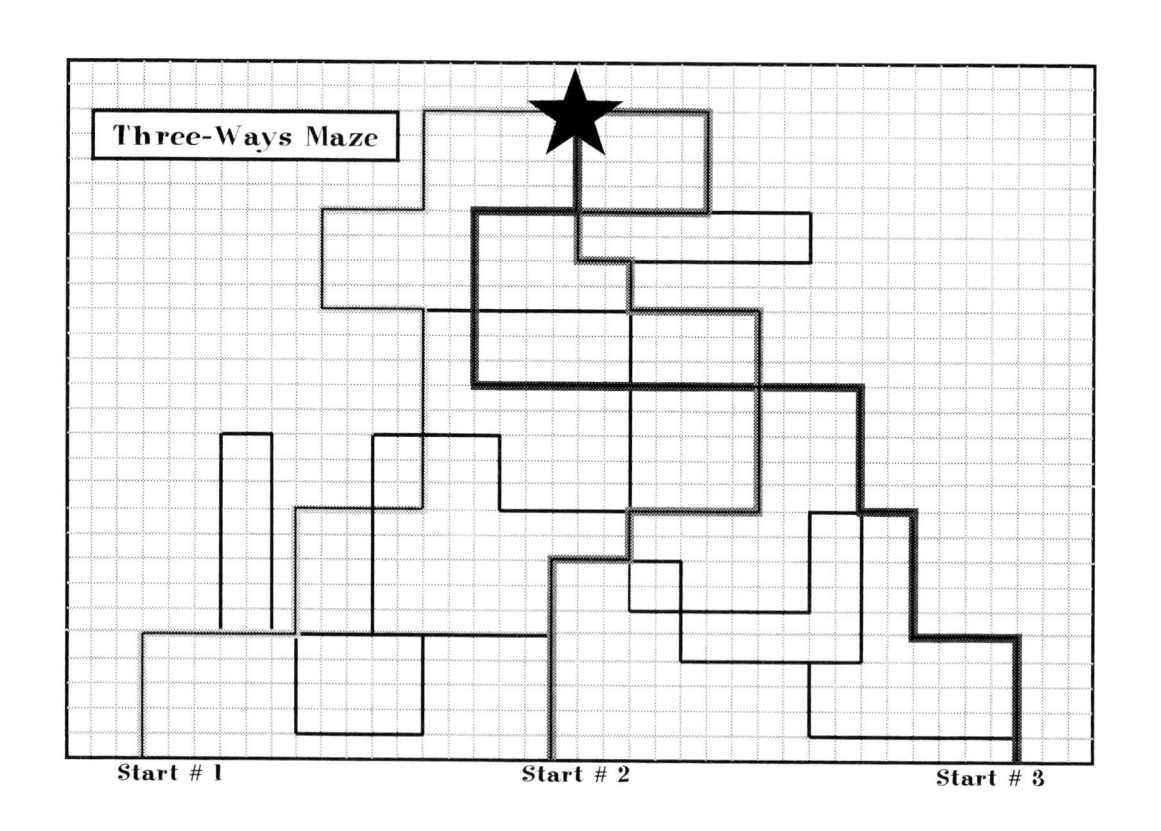

Three-Ways Maze

Start # 1   Start # 2   Start # 3

Secret Door

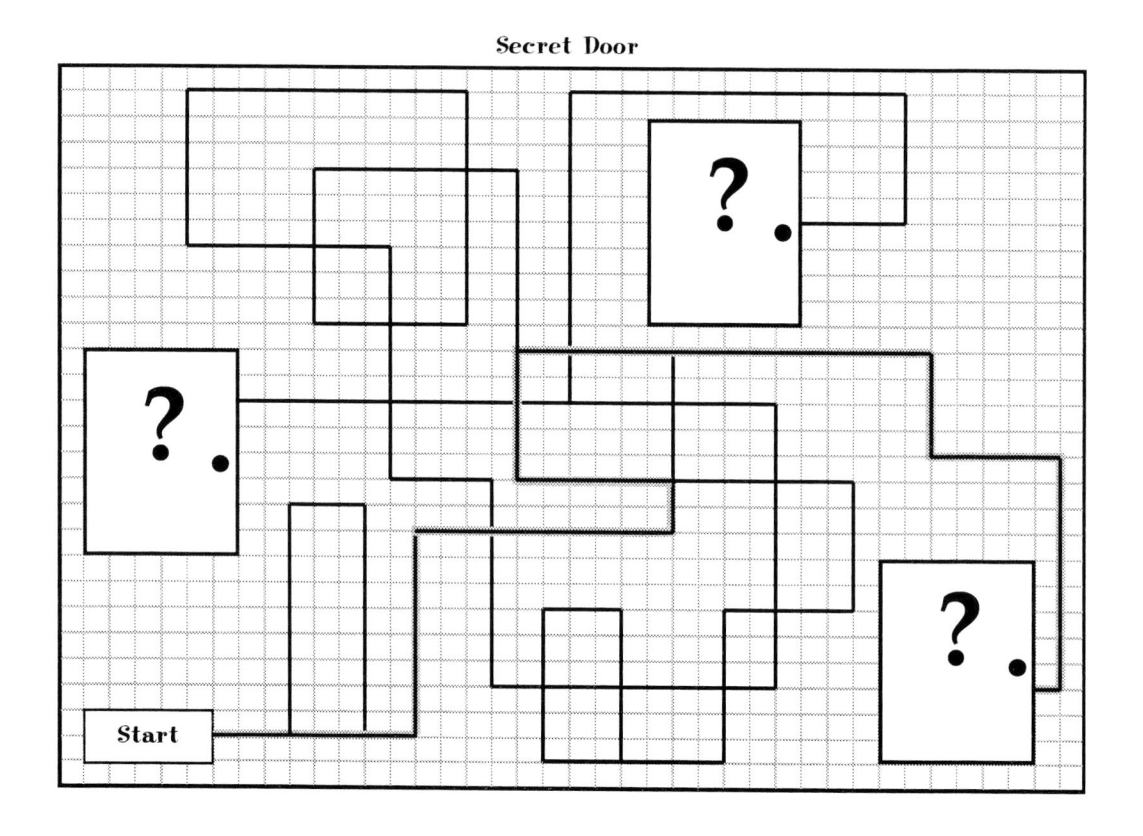

Start

APPENDIX

Glossary

Bilateral Integration - the ability to coordinate left and right sides of the body during activity (AOTA, 1994)

Body Awareness - receiving and differentiating sensory stimuli from inside and outside the body

Body Concept - identifying body parts by name (de Quirós and Schrager, 1979)

Body Division - notion that the body is anatomically and neurologically separated into right and left sides; separation of the body by planes of motion

Body Image - a mental image of the body that is modified by emotional and social influences as well as sensorimotor factors

Body Scheme - awareness of the the spatial relationships among body parts (AOTA, 1994)

Cognitive Map - a visual image of a landmark, location, destination or route

Cardinal Directions - North, South, East and West

Directional Concepts - concepts with spatial components such as in, out, under, over, up, down, top, bottom, front, back, forward, backward, left, right, far, near and the cardinal directions

Directional Confusion - the inability to interpret and apply directional concepts for functional use

Directional Coordinates - perpendicular lines arranged in a grid format that are referenced to the cardinal directions

Directional Language Concepts - words used to describe spatial components such as in, out, under, over, up, down, top, bottom, front, back, forward, backward, left, right, far, near and the cardinal directions

Directionality - projection of an internal sense of left and right onto external elements such as objects and locations

Extrapersonal Space - space outside the body

Fixed Reference Points - the cardinal directions: North, South, East and West

Form Constancy - the ability to identify forms and objects as the same when position, size or background has been altered (AOTA, 1994)

Frontal Plane - body plane dividing the body into front and back halves

Intrapersonal Space - space within the body

Laterality - using a preferred body side for a specialized task (AOTA, 1994); awareness of left and right body sides (Kephart, 1960)

Lateralization - process whereby hemispheres become specialized for a particular function

Left–Right Confusion - the inability to differentiate the left side of the body from the right side of the body

Orienteering - officially recognized sport of cross-country navigation using a map and a compass

Perceptual Processing - the ability to organize sensory input into meaningful patterns (AOTA, 1994)

Position in Space - determining the position of an object relative to the self (Schneck, 1996)

Postural Integration - interaction between the vestibular, proprioceptive and visual systems, coordinated by the cerebellum, emerging at three or four years of age (de Quirós and Schrager, 1979)

Praxis - the ability to plan a new motor response to an environmental demand (AOTA, 1994)

Proprioceptors - sensory receptors originating in muscles, joints and internal tissues that relay information about body position (AOTA, 1994)

Quadruped - developmental position in which the body is supported on hands and knees with the hips aligned over the knees and the shoulders aligned over the hands

Right–Left Discrimination - the ability to differentiate right from left (AOTA, 1994)

Sagittal Plane - body plane dividing the body into left and right halves

Sensorimotor Period - period of development described by Piaget during which learning occurs as a result of sensory input and motor response to that input

Sensory Awareness - receiving and differentiating sensory input (AOTA, 1994)

Sensory Processing - the ability to interpret sensory input (AOTA, 1994)

Somatodyspraxia - deficient motor planning associated with concurrent tactile and proprioceptive processing deficits (Parham and Mailloux, 1996)

Spatial Analysis and Planning - interpreting and organizing spatial information for functional use (Levine, 1991)

Spatial Operations - the ability to manipulate the position of objects mentally (AOTA, 1994)

Spatial Perception - organizing sensory information about the position of objects relative to the self or to other objects into meaningful patterns

Spatial Relations - determining the position of an object relative to the position of another object (AOTA, 1994)

Spatial Vision - the ability to locate objects in space through the visual system

Tactile System - sensory receptors located in the skin that interpret light touch, pressure, temperature, pain and vibration (AOTA, 1994)

Tall Kneeling - developmental position in which body is supported on knees with shoulders, hips and knees aligned

Topographical Orientation - the ability to locate an object or setting and determine a route leading to it (AOTA, 1994)

Transverse Plane - body plane dividing the body into top and bottom halves

Vestibular–Proprioceptive Feedback - information about body position originating from inner ear receptors in combination with information about body position originating from muscles, joints and internal tissues that occurs as a result of active movement

Vestibular–Proprioceptive System - sensory system interpreting stimuli originating from the inner ear, working in combination with the sensory system interpreting stimuli originating in muscles, joints and other internal tissues

Visual Perception - receiving and organizing visual stimuli into meaningful patterns

Wayfinding - the ability to find one's way in the environment

References

Abreau, B. C. *Physical Disabilities Manual.* New York: Raven Press, 1981.

Allen, A. S. and Clark, P.N. (Eds.), *Occupational Therapy for Children.* St. Louis: Mosby, 1985.

American Occupational Therapy Association. *Uniform Terminology for Occupational Therapy–Third Edition.* Rockville, MD: The American Occupational Therapy Association, Inc., 1994.

Anderson, S. *The Orienteering Book.* Mountain View, CA: Anderson World Inc., 1977.

Aquaro, M. B., et al. *OT Goals.* Tucson: Therapy Skill Builders, 1992.

Asher, I. E. *Occupational Therapy Assessment Tools: An Annotated Index–Second Edition.* Bethesda: The American Occupational Therapy Association, Inc., 1996.

Ayres, A. J. *Southern California Sensory Integration Tests–Manual.* Los Angeles: Western Psychological Services, 1979.

Ball, T. S. and Edgar, C. L. The effectiveness of sensory-motor training in promoting generalized body image development. *Journal of Special Education,* vol. 5, no. 8: 387-395 (1967).

Bundy, A. C. and Koomar, J. A. The Art and Science of Creating Direct Intervention from Theory. In Fisher, A. G., Murray, E. A. and Bundy A. C. (Eds.), *Sensory Integration: Theory and Practice.* Philadephia: F. A. Davis, 1991.

Clark, F., Clark, P. N. and Florey, L. A. Developmental Principles and Theories. In Allen, A. S. and Clark, P. N. (Eds.), *Occupational Therapy for Children.* St. Louis: Mosby, 1985.

Colarusso, R. P. and Hammill, D. D. *Motor-Free Visual Perception Test–Revised.* Novato: Academic Therapy Publications, 1995.

Cruickshank, W. M. and Hallahan, D. P. *Psychoeducational Foundations of Learning Disabilities.* Englewood Cliffs: Prentice-Hall, Inc., 1973.

Culp, R. E., Packard, V. N. and Humphry, R. Sensory motor versus cognitive perceptual training effects on the body concepts of preschoolers. *American Journal of Occupational Therapy,* vol. 34, no.4: 259-262 (1980).

de Quirós, J. B. and Schrager, O. L. *Neuropsychological Fundamentals in Learning Disabilities–Revised Edition.* Novato, CA: Academic Therapy Publications, 1979.

Fisher, A. G. Vestibular-Proprioceptive Processing and Bilateral Integration and Sequencing Deficits. In Fisher, A. G., Murray, E. A. and Bundy, A. C., (Eds.), *Sensory Integration: Theory and Practice.* Philadelphia: F.A. Davis, 1991.

Gardner, M. F. *Test of Visual-Perceptual Skills (Non-Motor).* Burlingame, CA: Psychological and Educational Publications, 1982.

Jordan, B. T. *Jordan Left–Right Reversal Test, Third Revised Edition.* Novato, CA: Academic Therapy Publications, 1990.

Kephart, N. C. *The Slow Learner in the Classroom.* Columbus, OH: Charles E. Merrill Publishing Co., 1960.

Knoblock, H. and Passaminick, B. *Gesell's Manual of Developmental Diagnosis–Revised.* New York: Harper and Row, 1980.

Laurendau, M. and Pinard, A. *Development of the Concept of Space in the Child.* New York: International University Press, 1970.

Levine, K. J. *Fine Motor Dysfunction: Therapeutic Strategies in the Classroom.* Tucson: Therapy Skill Builders, 1991.

Maloney, M., Ball, T. and Edgar, C. L. Analysis of the generalizability of sensory motor training. *American Journal of Mental Deficiency,* vol. 74: 458-469 (1970).

McMonnies, C. W. *Overcoming Left/Right Confusion and Reversals: A Classroom Approach.* North Sydney, Australia: Superior Educational Publications, 1991.

McVey, V. *The Sierra Club Wayfinding Book.* San Francisco: Sierra Club Books, 1989.

Mitchell, A. W. Theories of body scheme development. *Physical & Occupational Therapy in Pediatrics,* vol. 17, no. 4: 25-45 (1997).

Murray, E. A. Hemispheric Specialization. In Fisher, A. G., Murray E. A., and Bundy, A. C. (Eds.), *Sensory Integration Theory and Practice.* Philadelphia: F. A. Davis, 1991.

Nash, J. Your own personal adventure. *Diabetes Forecast,* vol. 48, no. 9: 42-49 (1995).

Parham, L. D. and Mailloux, Z. Sensory Integration. In Allen, A. S., Case-Smith, J. and Pratt, P. N. (Eds.), *Occupational Therapy for Children–Third Edition.* St. Louis: Mosby, 1996.

Roach, E. G. and Kephart. N. C. *The Purdue Perceptual-Motor Survey.* Columbus: Merrill, 1996.

Schneck, C. Visual Perception. In Allen, A. S., Case-Smith, J. and Pratt, P. N. (Eds.), *Occupational Therapy for Children–Third Edition.* St Louis: Mosby, 1996.

Sunal, C. S. Training program for kindergarten children identified as potentially perceptual motor disabled. *Reading Improvement,* vol. 15, no. 3: 208-214 (1978).

About the Author

Laura Sena, B.A., B.S., OTR/L, graduated from the University of New Mexico with degrees in clinical psychology, special education and studio art. Laura went on to study occupational therapy at the University of Washington. She returned to the Southwest and has practiced occupational therapy in a variety of settings for the last sixteen years. Laura currently works with children with learning disabilities and adults who are developmentally disabled in Santa Fe, New Mexico, where she lives with her husband, Phil, and children, Marie and Mark. In addition to *A Sense of Direction*, Ms. Sena is also the author of *Chalkboard Fun* published by Imaginart.